MW01104062

Squared Away

Squared Away is a literary presentation of factual information. Sometimes humorous, but always informative, *Squared Away* describes a powerful yet practical approach to shaping a healthier Whole Body future. These two words broaden our understanding of, and give us the ability to apply, the concepts that define the *Squared Away* approach to: acquiring an energetic, attractive and neutrally performing body structure.

Squared Away:

- Describes a well-aligned and pain-free body performance and appearance

- Defines the valid results of a scrupulously researched and personally-validated lifetime of investigations

- Expresses the body's rejuvenated and renewed body form and function

- Explains the intricate connections among the collective parts of the musculoskeletal system

- Creates a life sustaining atmosphere for improving, maintaining and specializing our body condition

Squared Away is larger than all its parts---a distinguished expression of knowledge and understanding that can bring exceptional results.

Squared Away

*Rejuvenate Your
Body Strength
and
Flexibility*

Mary L. Shuck, Ed.D.
In Collaboration With
John "Ed" Fellow, M.D.

Copyright © 2012 by Mary L. Shuck, Ed.D.
All rights reserved. No part of this book may
be reproduced in any form without written
permission from her. Printed in the United
States of America.

Author of Chapter 5: John "Ed" Fellow, M.D.
Illustrations: Barbara Nelson, Pat Rogondino
Cover Design: Pat Rogondino
Book Design and Production: Pat Rogondino

Legal Advisor:
Michael Hoisington, Attorney at Law
Higgs Fletcher & Mack LLP
401 West "A" Street, Ste. 2600
San Diego, CA 92101

Dedication

IN HONOR AND APPRECIATION
of
BARRY MCDONNELL

A True and Dedicated Teacher

This book is dedicated to Barry McDonnell, a man whom I have known and considered to be my friend for over thirty years. I have often referred to Barry as resembling the character Robert Duval played in the movie *Lonesome Dove*. Instead of a rifle, Barry carried a golf club, and rode in a car, not on a horse. But, both men had a code of ethics and a strong moral fiber that were inseparable. Neither one seemed to be hesitant about expressing his opinion. Nor were they short of words when telling someone to "get his/her act together."

Barry was also a wise and patient teacher. Through the years,

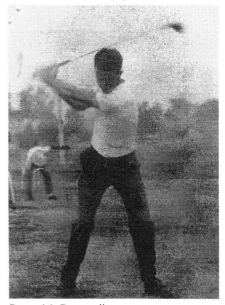

Barry McDonnell

I would watch him instructing young golfers at the Murrieta Valley Golf Range, where he was head pro and co-owner. One such golfer was Rickie Fowler—a long-time student—who would give to Barry his own professional goal by making the PGA tour.

I am sure that many of Barry's students still treasure some of Barry's short phrases of advice. I call them "Barryisms." He would repeat these one-liners over and over when teaching us about golf and how to play the game. Such remarks tend to stay with the learner because when a man of few words, with such timely perception and teaching talent speaks, we not only listen, but those words stay with us for a life time. I recall some that he said to me: "Mary, you think too much, or, …don't doubt yourself," or, "Keep that left hand going forward."

Barry's life-long friend and partner, Bill Teasdale, recalls some of these jewels: "The greatest strikers in history are self taught, this also confuses most golf instructors," also saying, "If you want more yardage, move up a set of tees."

Barry's advice to Rickie Fowler went something like…."That might be the one you roll in for the birdie." Barry was referring to a miss hit; when he said, … "just stay patient, Rick, …just go beat Old Man Par." His advice to would-be-advisors went something like… "stay out of his way, the little man will get it done."

Rick honors his friend saying, "Barry wasn't only a golf coach to me but a life coach and someone that I looked up to. Most everything I know and do on the golf course came from Big B (that's what I always called him)."

Barry died last year, 2011 on May 24th. I miss him every day.

Truly, this gentleman was exceptional in every sense of the word.

ABOUT THE AUTHOR

Early in life I realized that internal health and external appearances were inseparable. These are the fundamental concepts on which the Squared Away philosophy and approach to musculoskeletal Whole Body Health are based.

My credentials and background for writing this manuscript include:

- Degrees from the University of Southern California — B.S., M.S., Ed.D.

- CEO and Owner of Carefully Planned consulting company---training others for management and leadership responsibilities, also in writing and speaking skills

- Visiting Professor at Cal State University at Long Beach, CA

- Published, August, 1973, dissertation investigating Learning Theory and Human Behavior

- Supporting consultant, published by Time, Inc., *The 100 Events that Shaped America, Bicentennial Issue LIFE Special Report*

- Management and leadership responsibilities in the public sector, focused on training, developing, managing programs and theories to guide learning and instruction

- Augmenting these credentials is my life-long journey of pursuing scientific research and personally experimenting with physiological and biological practices. I have always appreciated having a sense of "feeling good" when knowing that I was physically fit and also looking like it

- Hosting seminars and guest speaker on above topics throughout thirty-plus years in the work place

Contents

Acknowledgements

Many individuals have made this publication possible. Some are aware of their contributions and others came to my attention through resources I studied. I have great appreciation for the current scientists as well as those who in the past investigated and wrote about anatomical, physiological and biological sciences. Their work is remarkable and always thought provoking.

To those with whom I've had close association during this project, my contact with each of you has been priceless. Les has been a very tolerant and caring husband—adjusting his life style to mine during these three-and-a-half years.

Dr. John "Ed" Fellow, is a collaborator and contributor to the content in Squared Away. His chapter on imbalances gives you a sampling of how a skilled sports medicine specialist sees and treats musculoskeletal injuries. During Ed's twenty-five years of practicing sports medicine and over thirteen years at Scripps Clinic, Rancho Bernardo, CA, he has experienced many professional accomplishments. Focusing on clinical orthopedics and solving problems or resolving patients' medical issues, have provided him with a tremendous sense of self-worth and brought him many honors.

My wonderful friend, Barbara Nelson, has been exceptionally generous, providing moral support and encouragement over the past three years. She has spent many hours applying her finely tuned editing skills and artistic creativity to this manuscript. Barbara and her husband, Bryant, are artists. Barbara created the figures for the cover.

Pat Rogondino's creative thought and wide breadth of knowledge about formatting manuscripts for printing, speaks for itself. Pat is best described as a thoroughly honorable and intelligent woman who just happens to be my neighbor, a close friend and a creative photographer. Pat is especially gifted in her profession— production graphics specialist. Her artistic creations masterfully interpreted the messages intended to make Squared Away an attractive and treasured manuscript.

I am particularly grateful to Don Byrd, a highly skilled golf professional at San Luis Rey Downs, Bonsall, CA. Don has an eloquent mastery of many languages—all English—but geared to speaking to each player's golfing ability. During the past five years, he has helped me make adjustments in my golf swing to fit the changes occurring in my muscles and body posture. His knowledge of how body mechanics relate to the individual's golfing ability has brought him respect and appreciation from his students and fellow golf professionals. It is wonderful when you can have such gifts in one golf instructor. I have had that privilege twice.

Kelly James, HHP, a massage therapist. had an early interest in the Squared Away approach. Several years ago, we looked into the idea that imbalances can be improved through massage therapy. She prescribed programs for a few of her students and found they had relief from muscle irritations when following the program for only a few weeks. Over the years, I have lost contact with Kelly. I hope she is doing well.

The Scripps La Jolla, Physical Therapy Clinic is well known for helping sportsmen and sportswomen as well as the not-so-normal people, correct their musculoskeletal problems. I had direct contact with a capable young man, Alan Ferrarelli, Manager of Rehabilitation Services. Alan mentioned in his memo to me, January 30, 2009, that there is a need for people to become more aware of their own anatomy, and that my reference to keeping the body aligned during exercises was one of the basic principles of exercise therapy. I was also a student at the headquarters of the Egosque Method, San Diego, CA, where I received fine professional care from the skilled staff.

A woman named Kat Folger came into my life about two years ago. Kat has a plethora of professional credentials, is fully certified by L.B.D.C., and is an accomplished instructor and respected leader in teaching Pilates and yoga. She is a Creative Exercise Specialist for pain relief, instructing physical conditioning based on the theory that proposes — our muscles were designed to perform every body movement necessary when the body structure fits the neutral anatomical body structure.

Two highly professional editors, Rosalie & Michael Pakenham, twice reviewed my manuscript. Each review was skillfully edited and their suggestions were most appreciated. I am grateful to them for their encouragement and recommendations.

Trenton Niemi improved my awareness and understanding of how our senses interact, and can accelerate changes we want to make in our musculoskeletal system. Trenton has a master's degree from San Diego State University in Exercise Physiology, and is presently an instructor at the University of Hawaii, Maui Campus in physiology and anatomy. It was a pleasure getting acquainted with such an intelligent and personable young professional.

As I recall the past, I can also appreciate the Great Creator for helping me learn, then share, my learning with others.

Blessed is the man who finds wisdom,
the man who gains understanding.
Proverbs 3:13

YOU FIRST

Ask Yourself

■ Are my skeletal muscles in need of improvement?

■ If so, how bad is their condition?

■ How can I fix them?

Squared Away Relates to You

You may be asking, "What does this book have to do with me?" The answer is *"Everything."* This is a book about gaining information that puts you in control of your body: strength, appearance and performance. After all, who is not interested in having a body showing some pizzazz, while presenting a strikingly confident and healthy body condition? The years that I have spent, personally experimenting with and studying about, physiological and biological theories and practices, have given me a broad spectrum for developing the Squared Away approach to everyday physiological fitness and Whole Body Health practices.

Maybe you are thinking that there is nothing wrong with your posture, and the way you move. This is exactly what many have said before coming in contact with the Squared Away Self-investigations. So, before you put the book down, finish reading these pages.

The Book Works for You

You will appreciate the format and language that have (a) synthesized (b) organized and (c) calmed-down the rather detailed vocabulary often used when addressing these topics. The content goes directly to providing you with exceptional information, relating to you, how you look and move → in your every day life style. Read this book with the intention of changing some beliefs and assumptions that you have long held dear about being physically fit. Maybe you will no longer be believing what you think.

I have always appreciated having a sense of "feeling good" when knowing that I was physiologically fit and looking like it.

Squared Away Defined

The term, Squared Away, has been interpreted in many ways. I consider it as a quality way-of-life. It is also referred to as a body condition that represents an evenly aligned and naturally performing body structure. I really like the way some military personnel interpret the idea of being Squared Away when they are describing those who have "Their Act Together." Who doesn't want that?

Be prepared to learn how to *improve* skeletal muscles needing rehabilitation, and *stabilizing* those that are performing efficiently and effectively. Squared Away does that for you.

1

STRAIGHT TALK

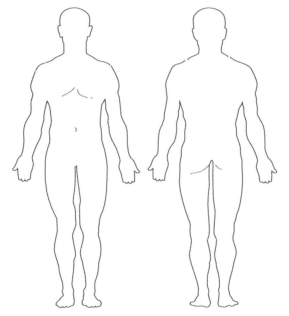

Neutral anatomical body structure

A Day to Remember

When we look in the mirror, perhaps we do not always like what we see. About five years ago while standing in front of my mirror, I could hardly recognize the body structure being reflected. How in the world had my body gotten into this irregular condition? Shoulders were unevenly positioned with one another, and my hips somehow seemed to be twisted. The image that I was looking at certainly had no resemblance to an evenly shaped and elegantly aligned, Squared Away body physique. What was going on here? In the past, I thought I looked fairly well-aligned; and I certainly

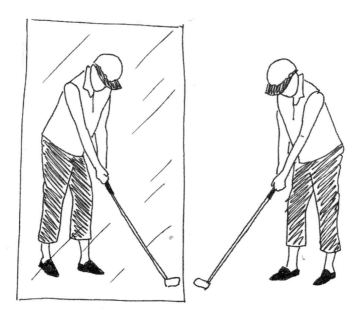

felt physiologically fit. So, how come my body resembled a train wreck? Maybe you have experienced a similar awakening, or would like to know how to move without muscle tension or restrictions. You are in the right place to gain information about improving your musculoskeletal system. Squared Away will help you to do just that.

Personally Speaking

Squared Away is *not* a book about golf, rather it came about because I play the game of golf. Actually, it began the day I stood in front my mirror, following my golf pro's suggestion that I should see for myself how I was pulling the club face off target.

I knew I had some irregularities in my back and shoulders, but outside of some nagging pain in my shoulders and a few limitations in movement, these structural conditions seemed to have little effect on my participation in daily or physical fitness activities. I certainly had not noticed the gradual deterioration in my body alignment — thus performance and appearance — that was slowly getting worse. It is difficult for us to recognize the muscle changes taking place in our physiological and anatomical body systems when we look at them every day.

Many of us go through our daily lives unnecessarily putting up with limitations in our ability to move naturally. You probably have recognized others who are plagued with either early or advanced

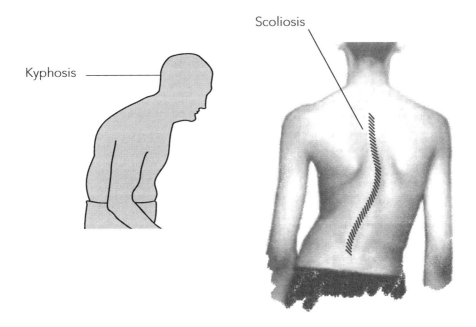

Kyphosis

Scoliosis

stages of two very common skeletal muscle problems: *kyphosis* and *scoliosis*. **Kyphosis** is a convex curvature of the spine (collapsed chest, head is forward, shoulders are rounded) and **scoliosis** (asymmetrical deviations of the spine, shoulders and hip).

My response to dealing with these two conditions was to build, and maintain, strong and flexible muscles that would form good balance and performance. It was certainly clear that my musculoskeletal system needed an entirely different approach than the one I had been following. Getting my shoulders and spinal column more evenly aligned would involve not only restructuring, but somehow, getting my muscles to relax and perform with more flexibility. My emphasis on strength and discipline had to go. I needed to find a way out of this confusion.

This is where you, the reader, enter the picture. Be aware, that these opportunities are available to you when you pay closer attention to your body alignment (posture) and take more seriously the changes that are appearing in your body structure.

> **You can more easily improve postural misalignments that are disrupting normal skeletal muscle performance, and find out how to return atypical muscle movements to normal performance without losing your patience in the long process.**

Although this book is not a personal memoir nor strictly a self-help publication, I have used a personal event to introduce you to the importance of paying proper attention to our body posture. The incident I had in front of my mirror, became a turning-point in my life. Up to that time, my study and personal participation in exercise and therapy programs were not crucial. That casual attitude changed rather abruptly.

I had some unknowns to resolve and time was of the essence. Ultimately, several years later, I would find help for restoring much of my atypical body posture, thus body alignment. In addition, I would also discover that, in all probability, most of these deviations could have been prevented.

Fortunately, I did not have to start from scratch to pursue the cause and affect relationships between my imbalances and misshaped skeletal muscles. Having a life-long interest in the human body physiological, anatomical and biological sciences had prepared me well for facing this dilemma. The years spent conducting my own personal investigations, and participating in numerous physiological, body movement practices, were a wonderful asset during the last three-and-a-half years. Being familiar with the anatomical structures of muscle, bone and tissue, was not the problem. Rather, I needed to understand how to appropriately move specific body parts so I could bring them back to their normal positions—which would then improve their performance.

Self-Awareness is Important

If you have been looking in the mirror to see
if you might have some body parts that look a
bit irregular, take a bow. Such behavior will get
you far. Self-awareness comes about by paying
close attention to your postural condition,
and the way your body moves. Keeping them
performing properly will help you recognize
how wide the range of interference can be,
and once identified, how to properly make
corrections and eliminate sources that cause them. Every chapter in
the text helps you cultivate and refine these understandings.

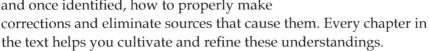

Be mindful that it has taken your body, the number of years
you are old, to arrive at its current body condition. Therefore,
making changes in the body structure will not take place over night.
Squared Away methods can help you circumvent unworthy pursuits
by offering you a direct route for improving your posture while
increasing your body *flexibility* and *strength*. Becoming dedicated to
such accomplishments is one thing. But, the skills that you hold dear
will be those developed when making the Squared Away principles
work for you.

Various degrees of interference occur regularly in our muscles
and surrounding tissue. Such disruptions can cause a whole range
of skeletal muscle problems — from mild, to moderate, to severe.
These events include those occurring during our every day activities
as well as those considered to be unusual. Some will be short-term
while others will be more permanent.

Not all of our injuries can be easily recognized or treated by the
novice. Professional help will be needed for certain skeletal structure
imperfections. The Squared Away approach provides you with
information so you can improve unnatural postural and alignment
problems. Most of us have experienced some events in our past,
which without our recognizing their impact, have left their mark
on our body's performance and/or appearance. Possibly you have
some thoughts about physical maintenance that are interfering with
your body's normal form and function. Here are some common
"detractors" to consider. Are any of them familiar to you?

ABCs of Muscle Performance Disruptions

A. Accidents-minor or major

B. Bad habits practiced over long periods of time

C. Coping with various illnesses and previous medical procedures

D. Delaying treatment

E. Excessive expectations of muscle performance

F. Favoring healing body parts during recovery

G. Guessing rather than knowing about reliable information

Truly, mistakes are held to a minimum when our thoughts are realistically sound, and our Self-activating Skills are working. We can react with confidence when we understand the cause-and-affect relationships between imbalances and body performance.

Knowledge and Information Work Well Together

Getting involved with the Squared Away approach is a major undertaking because it involves Whole Body Health. This means that self-managing your thoughts, and staying focused on them, enables you to have direct connections between your physicality and reliable information. You are introduced to techniques and information to use when making judgments on the qualifications of those giving advice as well as critiquing the calibre of advice being given.

When you have good information to guide your decisions and actions, you will *not* have to go through life coping with pain, poor posture and unattractive postural alignment. Such conditions include poor muscle form and function that are painful most of the time, and those that register pain or stress when pressure is applied to them. Staying alert to our body condition, is definitely intelligent behavior.

Be reminded that Squared Away focuses on improving postural misalignments by making changes in skeletal muscles. The approach does *not* have relevance to correcting skeletal structures other than moving the muscles that are attached to them.

In the text, I use the term "hot spots" when referring to pain that we experience when pressure is applied to our skeletal muscles.

6

Hidden agenda refers to extended areas that are affected by tight and stressed tissue that remain unnoticed until pressure is applied. These are the signals we often discount, believing them to be unimportant and not needing our attention.

Validation of Book Content

Opinionaire

When starting to write Squared Away, I asked a diverse group of people to give their opinions about the Squared Away concepts. My sources included a medical doctor, physical therapists, school teachers, students and professionals in various fields of physical health. I knew that I was on the right track when their informative comments, made on the Opinionaire, confirmed conclusions that I had drawn about self-assessment. This is an opportunity to discover misalignments previously undetected and recognize those that have become unnaturally fixed in our musculoskeletal system. The Squared Away approach made sense to this group because it has authentic grounding in research that can be applied to activities in our daily lives. A sample of my Opinionaire is in the back of the book.

Testimonials of Participants

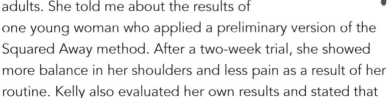

Several years ago, I was a patient of a fine massage therapist who became interested in the investigations I was making to correct my misalignments. Kelly James, HHP. treated both male and female adults. She told me about the results of one young woman who applied a preliminary version of the Squared Away method. After a two-week trial, she showed more balance in her shoulders and less pain as a result of her routine. Kelly also evaluated her own results and stated that the pain and stiffness in her lower back were minimized after practicing exercises for only two weeks.

The remainder of this chapter provides information about imbalances, and explains fundamentals on which Squared Away is based. Information throughout the text addresses ways of properly moving one's muscles—whether being *maintained, improved* or *specialized*.

Imbalances, Misalignments and Definitions

Before we proceed, two terms need clarification. In this book, the meanings of muscle imbalances and misalignments are interchanged. These terms describe irregular muscle conditions and their effects on our skeletal posture. *Random House Webster's Unabridged Dictionary* defines muscle imbalances as faulty muscular or glandular conditions, whereas misalignments simply mean being improperly aligned. I have taken liberty with these two terms when referring to uneven or irregular muscle and skeletal conditions that take place when normal muscle performance is disturbed. Therefore, for the purpose of this text, muscles and body posture are considered to have both traits—being imbalanced and misaligned.

Staying Current

Imbalances are not skin deep nor are they easily eliminated. There is much to be done after noticing that our posture could use a little correction. Maybe you have some rather "stiff" body parts, or you have noticed that picking things up off the floor has recently become a major event. Actually, these seemingly slight irritations are really quite serious, and in need of your attention. We are quickly reminded that uneven posture is more than skin deep. In order to correct them, we need to look beyond the effect and focus on the cause. Changing them does *not* happen by doing something silly like repeating my friend's solution. She calmly removed all the large mirrors in her house, except for one hand mirror. People are interesting, aren't they?

Checking Reality: Three Tenets Do the Job

There are three conspicuous truths that describe misshaped body parts. Adopting these pronouncements brings you onto common ground with the experts.

The First Tenet proposes that undetected misalignments, possibly remaining unrecognized for years, allow our muscles to become fixed in unnatural positions. When some occur slowly, they are not only difficult to recognize, but because other body parts have tried to cope, a plethora of misshaped and poorly performing body parts can occur.

The Second Tenet claims that musculoskeletal misalignments are quite common. Regardless of our physical strength or level of physical discipline, unnatural form and function in our musculoskeletal system is quite ordinary. Do not be surprised if you find unnatural body performance and appearances in your *skeletal* muscles.

The Third Tenet tells us that every body movement affects our posture, especially when frequently repeated. Even the slightest repetition of a body movement, over time, can have an impact on our postural alignment form and function. We can claim to have well-grounded contact with our musculoskeletal system, only when we also have a healthy kinetic relationship with its component parts. Being able to repeat the proper kinesthesia—proper sensation in our muscles—gives us the power to control them. We are talking about the power to *improve* and *maintain* natural conditions, or *specialize* to achieve more exceptional performance of our muscle movements.

Taking ownership of these Tenets secures a firm foundation for evaluating our body condition. By making daily use of them, you can advance your level of self-awareness to include a willingness to search, find and correct portions of your body structure. You have probably decided by now that dismissing and/or minimizing irregularities in our musculoskeletal system, is not a good idea.

Three Important Questions

- Do I have some skeletal muscles in need of improvement?

- If I do, how bad is the condition?

- How can I fix them?

Making a habit of asking and having answers to these questions will help you to stay on target as you participate in the activities requested of you, especially in the next several chapters.

Your Future has Potential

Throughout the text, I will be tenacious about encouraging you to elevate your self-awareness technique and to make use of the information printed on these pages. With the right amount of attention given to your reflections in the mirror, you can be the proud owner of a more naturally positioned body, representing a more attractive image.

If this seems overwhelming because already, you have "too many demands" from "too many people" — stay right here. Reading this book will help you dissolve defenses against taking action, and improve your existence by enhancing and stabilizing your body alignment. These are important incentives for adjusting old behaviors and out-of-date thinking as well as installing reliable practices. Let us see if the program I designed for reconfiguring my body posture and muscle composition, can affect yours in the same positive ways.

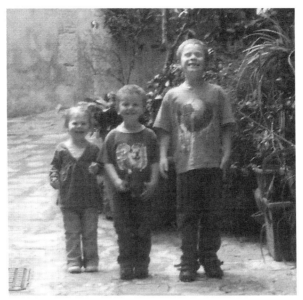

Left to right: Gwendolyn, Clayton, Case

Before leaving this chapter, take notice of these two photographs. The first one shows three children visiting Capalbio, Italy, in 2010. You probably have similar pictures of children showing how straight and evenly structured our bodies are when we are young.

Surfer in the United States

Although this illustration does not give you the "full monte" of the neutral body condition, you can see how the head, shoulders and hips are aligned even on a body board.

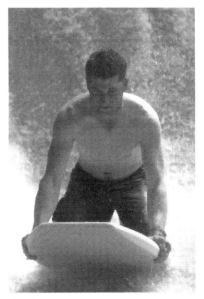

Philip

2

SETTING THE STAGE FOR ACQUIRING INFORMATION

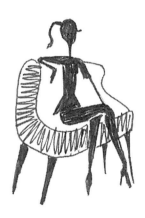

Accepting the Inevitable

I think we can agree that knowing as much as we can about our physicality will enable us to get the best results when trying to answer questions about our physical form and function. The next two chapters will help you discover some interesting facts about your particular body structure and performance. After all, one never knows what will be discovered from close scrutiny.

Self-Activating Skills

Help us obtain priceless intelligence and information about our physiological and biological status

Through our senses of touch and sight we gain maximum understanding of our muscle flexibility and strength.

Sensation of the position and movement of our body parts, is called kinesthesia. Combining your senses of feeling (touch) and sight with a reliable self-discovery process will deliver first-hand information to you. We use such sensitivity as we evaluate and manage our physiological body structure. Chapter Eleven goes into specific ways we use our senses. But, for now, you will be finding out about your body condition, by developing a daily routine involving self-awareness and self-assessment practices. For instance, "where" in your musculoskeletal system are muscles that are sensitive to pressure or are showing signs of irregular movements or positions? Do you know "when" or "how" these changes occurred?

Misshaped postural deviations are precursors to potential accidents and other health issues. You will be taking huge strides toward answering the first question, Do I have some skeletal muscles in need of repair? Although at this juncture you are *not* ready to deal with the other two questions, *How bad are the muscle imbalances* and *How can I fix them?* you are ready to find out if atypical muscle conditions are present. That is where we are right now. So let us find out.

Locating, Marking and Recording Body Points of Shoulder, Hip and Forehead

As you prepare to find your body point locations, take advantage of what you know about the Three Tenets that were described in Chapter One. Reflecting on their content can help reduce the anxiety you might have about the self-discovery process — reminding us that no one is perfect — these are guidelines that persevere throughout the

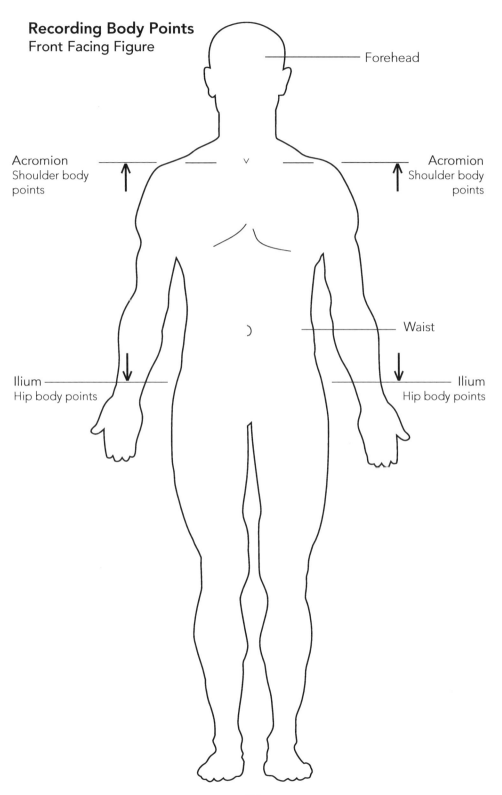

Recording Body Points
Front Facing Figure

Forehead

Acromion
Shoulder body points

Acromion
Shoulder body points

Waist

Ilium
Hip body points

Ilium
Hip body points

text. Using them at this time will serve you well. I have restated them here for your convenience.

> **It is possible for misalignments to go undetected for periods of time**
>
> **Most of us have experienced misalignments**
>
> **Even the slightest movement of our muscles contributes to muscle composition therefore, performance.**

Staying tuned into fluctuations within the musculoskeletal system is never ending, but is easily managed when you have the right skills to do so.

Finding and Marking your five body points: one on each hip and shoulder, and one on your forehead

This is a two-person project so have fun with it. Someone will need to be available to help you locate and record your **body points**. This half of the process sets the stage for taking your body measurements which are described in Chapter Three. But, let us not get the cart before the horse.

You can expect to get the best results from your self-assessment when you have all of your tools readily available: **(1)** a piece of chalk or a marking pen to mark your **body points** and **(2)** a pencil for recording on the figure provided. Wearing light clothing is also in order, and if possible, be close to a full-length mirror.

Locating and marking these areas prepare you for moving directly on to Chapter Three and completing your self-assessments. Hang in there, your time will be well-spent. You will be working from → your shoulders to → your waist to → your hips.

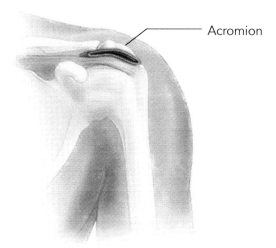

Acromion

Shoulder Body Points

Refer to the ilium and acromion Illustrations to help you locate **shoulder** and **hip body points**. Finding the acromion is the hardest part, but you will be able to do so by closely following these directions.

■ Stand with your back to your partner who will be locating the top of your scapula (shoulder blades) with fingertips and then following it out to where it connects with the shoulder joint. This can be felt when moving the fingertips about ½ of an inch away from the scapula and moving up toward the crest of the shoulder. You will feel a recessed area and then one more elevated as you move up to the top of the shoulder and are applying just a little pressure.

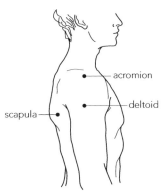

scapula
acromion
deltoid

This raised bone, that is closer to the neck and in front of the body, is the acromion. If you are unable to locate the acromion, find a spot on one shoulder and mark the same location on the other shoulder. Make these markings on the figure to record your **shoulder body points**.

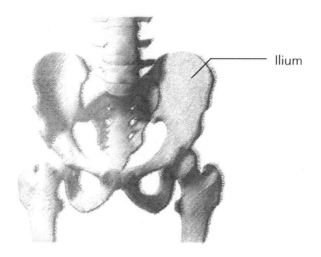

Ilium

Hip Body Points

Use the same preparations as before, and take notice of the iliac illustration.

- Working one side at a time, cup your hand so that your right hand is on your right hip with thumbs on the hip bone and fingers stretching back toward the buttocks. Slide thumb along hip bone away from your spine. Before it starts to curve down (inferiorly) you will feel the highest point on the bone surface. Use chalk or marking pen to make small markings on each hip, known as your **hip body points**. Mark your figure accordingly.

Forehead Body Point

- Mark center of your forehead as well as on the Front-facing figure.

Interpreting Your Findings

Are you congratulating yourself because all measured body points are within the one-half inch range when comparing each side of your body with the other? I congratulate you too. But, we need to finish the self-assessment before closing the book. Make sure that you go immediately to Chapter Three because you will be using these five body points.

3

SELF-ASSESSMENT
LOOKING DEEPER

Basics for Self-assessment

Self-assessment fills the gap between uncertainty and making appropriate choices by increasing what you know about your body condition and performance. In this chapter you will complete your self-assessment by taking measurements to guide you through the chapters that follow, especially when tattooing your practice mat and choosing your exercise regimen. Depending on the results that come to light, you will be taking charge of repairing (improving) maintaining and/or enhancing (specializing) your muscle performance. How do you like the sound of that?

Recognizing Muscle Conditions

In most instances, skeletal muscles will perform when in one of three conditions: (1) *atypical*—or unnaturally aligned or stressed— (2) *maintaining* a neutral body condition or (3) *specializing* when training for advanced performance. Before undertaking muscle treatments, it is important to know the status of your skeletal muscles so you can treat them properly.

Remember that skeletal muscles can continue to perform when in any of the three performance levels.

Skeletal muscles are remarkable body tissue; they often continue to perform, seemingly in normal fashion, even when they are abnormally positioned in *atypical* condition such as being under stress or experiencing other irregular conditions. You have read about my personal missteps with this situation. Of course, when in the *maintenance* status, we are keeping our muscles normalized, treating them with respect and intelligent consideration. *Specialized* status is just that. Muscles are trained to perform exceptionally as in dance, yoga, gymnastics, practicing advanced levels of Pilates, etc. Professionals who skate, golf and master other sports have also required their muscles to become **specialized**. Skeletal muscles have unbelievable stamina and performance capabilities, and when combined with the endurance capacity of the tissue that attaches them to bone, we are talking Rolls-Royce performance and endurance.

Even under severe circumstances our skeletal muscles continue contracting and providing us with instantaneous "up-dates" on their

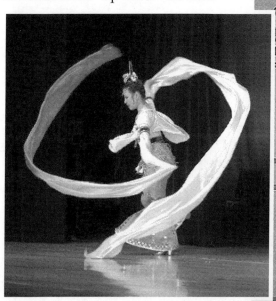

Lisa is a professional dancer, trained in China and continues to perform there every year.

condition. Discussions in later chapters refer to the influence the brain has on providing such enduring physiological and anatomical information. Your Self-activating Skills, coupled with knowledge gained from the Self-assessment Instruments, are only a part of the Squared Away "Quick Response" to Whole Body Health, especially when treating the musculoskeletal system.

Self-Assessment Has Personality

I am proud to show you these photographs of my friend, Bryant Nelson, who has personalized the Squared Away self-assessment process. He has translated information about his body alignment into real life existence. It is quite obvious that he has been dedicated to training his muscles to perform naturally. I am sure that you have noticed he has slight variances from the neutral anatomical ideal, but his body structure is certainly close to it.

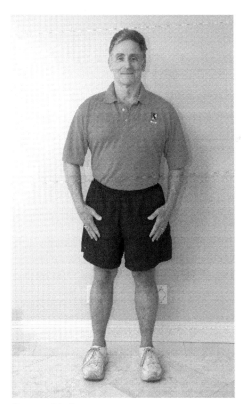

Bryant Nelson

Preparations _Before_ Beginning Body Measurements

General Directions

1. Technique for Taking a Stance

Your stance for each measurement should be as follows—
while looking straight ahead and breathing naturally, place
your feet only 3–4 inches apart, with arms hanging at your
side, and palms facing the side of your body. Be sure you
are free-standing so that no body part is touching any wall or
leaning against any object.

2. Technique for String Placement

Your partner should be facing you and holding the weighted
string slightly away from your **body point**, but directly in front
of it. Once you have started taking your measurements do not
readjust your stance. You want to see if various parts of your
body structure deviate from body point markings on each side
of the string (bi-lateral alignment).

3. Technique for Taking Measurements

Use a tape measure to stretch between
body points. Hold it firmly in your hands
and pull it taut between each of the
two markings. The person taking the
measurements may need to stand on a chair
to keep the tape from sagging.

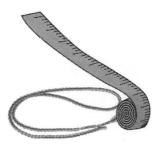

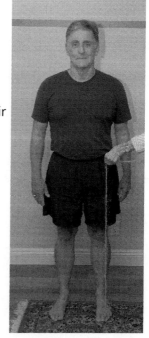

4. Materials Needed

The same preparations should be made for taking body measurements as those you used to locate **body points**. You definitely need someone to help you take and record your measurements. In addition, some readers purchase a posture or skeletal chart, and hang it on an adjoining wall to help them stay aligned during this fact-finding activity. This is a good idea. However, you can substitute by stretching a 40 inch long strip of tape on the wall parallel to the floor about six feet off the floor surface. Standing in front of this even line becomes a reliable point-of-reference when measuring your three body positions—FRONT (anterior), SIDES (lateral), and BACK (posterior).

Using a camera or cell phone for taking pictures is optional, but also quite helpful. In addition, you will need a measuring tape, yard stick (if possible) 2 lengths of string, a weight of some kind and of course, a very good friend. One string should be long enough to stretch from forehead to ankle with a weight on one end. To keep the string stable, attach a heavy object or use a plumb bob so the string can hang freely and straight. The shorter string should be long enough to reach around your hips and chest.

Front-Facing Upper Body Observations

Using the figure on the next page, you will be marking some arm measurements. Begin your self-assessment process by observing your body when looking in the mirror. This is simply a casual observation of your body posture, made without measurements, noticing how your shoulders and hips align.

Technique and Recording

Using the Stance for Each Measurement previously described, be sure that you are looking straight ahead, breathing naturally, feet only 3–4 inches apart, arms are hanging at your side and palms toward your body, and no body part is touching any wall or object. Now, notice the area where your arms are no longer touching your side, and where they are again resting against your hips—maybe near your wrists. This open space or "window" may resemble a triangle-like shape, where each arm stops touching the side and is again resting against it. They may not or may not be the same. Record what you see.

A Natural Body Structure

When each "window" or "triangle- opening" has the same shape, the alignment of your upper torso, shoulders in particular, is showing similar positions. In other words, the triangles drawn, showing how your arms hang from your shoulders, will indicate that one shoulder is **not** in front of the other, and the hips are **not** unevenly positioned. Being aware of such conditions is part of "today's information" to be used when making changes in your muscular form and function.

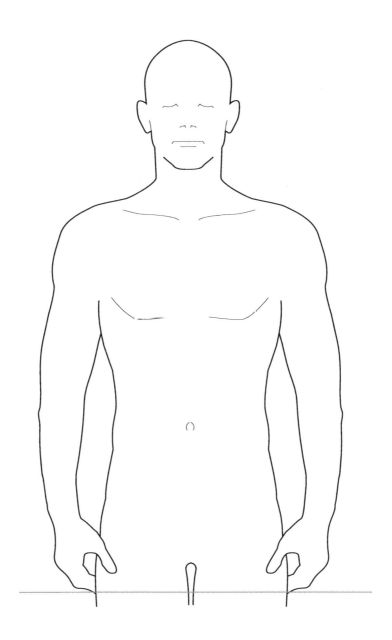

Taking Front-Facing Body Measurements

Technique and Recording

Stand in front of the mirror using the same directions as above, partner holds the string opposite forehead, and without touching any body part, the plumb bob falls to just above floor. Record the line on the figure and also sketch the atypical areas where parts of your body are uneven such as, one hip is farther from the center line than its partner, etc.

A Natural Body Structure

An evenly-shaped body structure will have the string falling from forehead body point, down past jugular or clavicular notch, then down past the center of the navel, past the top point of the pelvis and coming to rest just short of the floor surface, equal distance between the feet. See illustration.

Taking Other Measurements of Your Front-Facing Body Structure

Technique and Recording

Using string or measuring tape, as you stretch it between your various body parts, record on the lines provided.

Line A — Beginning at **center** of clavicular notch, lengthen string out to each **shoulder body point**. Record your measurements on figure. Repeat on other side.

Line B — Beginning at **shoulder body points** and measuring down to waist, record distance to waist on each LEFT and RIGHT side.

Line C — Use the same directions to record distances from **shoulder body points** to **hip body points**.

Line D — Partner holds shorter string around your hip area, having it pass directly over each **hip body point** when encircling the body. Draw a line indicating the path the string followed when being strung across each **hip body point**. Does the string, when wrapped, indicate variances in hip alignments?

Line E — Measure waist in the same fashion. Record path the string follows when stretched around the waist.

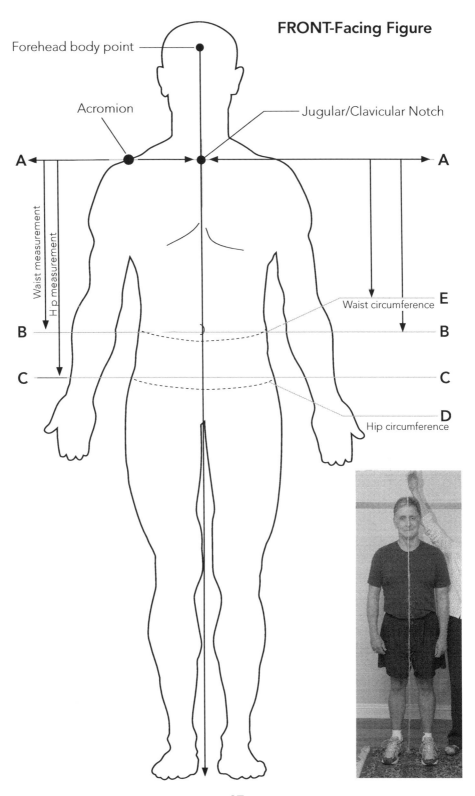

FRONT-Facing Figure

Forehead body point

Acromion

Jugular/Clavicular Notch

A — A

Waist measurement

H p measurement

Waist circumference — E

B — B

C — C

D

Hip circumference

Side-Facing Body Measurements

Side-Facing Figures

Technique and Recording

Use lines F to record both sides on each of the SIDE-Facing figures (next page.)

F — Your partner should be facing the side of your body and holding weighted string away from the body and opposite the **forehead body point**, with the plumb bob falling just above the floor and just forward of the ankle bone. The string-line may not pass directly through the shoulder points, so draw what your see on the LEFT and RIGHT SIDE-Facing Body Figures shown by the free falling string line-pattern.

A Natural Body Structure

The weighted string should fall freely, not touching the body as it passes alongside the earlobe, past the acromion crest and down alongside of rib cage, coming to rest just forward of the lateral ankle bone and above the floor surface. The body structure should be evenly positioned as in the illustration.

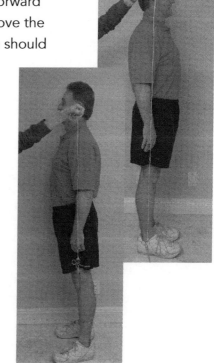

Line F — Holding short string opposite **shoulder body point**, let string free fall to waist and record distance to waist on each figure.

Line G — Following the same directions, measure to the hips.

SIDE-Facing Figure

RIGHT-SIDE Facing Figure

LEFT-SIDE Facing Figure

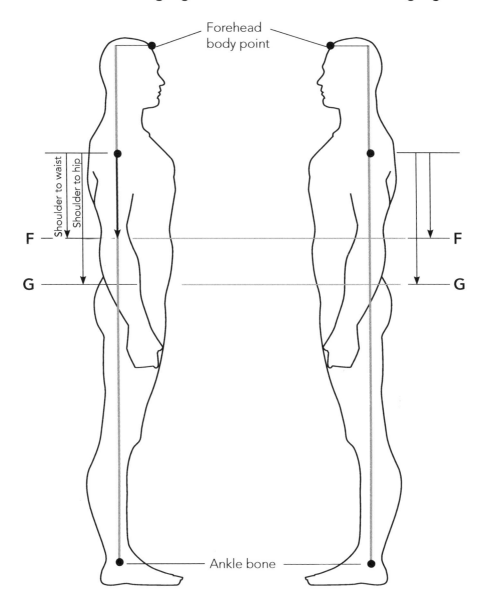

Use lines F and G to record measurements from shoulder body point to → waist F and to → hip G.

Record string path. It may not pass directly through shoulder body points. Record what you see.

Back-Facing Body Measurements

Posterior Body

Technique and Recording

You will be making your own lines on this figure as you take a stance 180 degrees from the FRONT- Facing Figure. Notice any unnatural positions of body structure. As you record what you see, you may need to draw on the figure in order to show where the two sides of the body are uneven. For instance, you may need to show where one shoulder is higher than the other or where one leg or foot turns out more than the other, etc.

A Natural Body Structure

Without the string touching the body, the string should fall freely from the center of the back of the head, passing along center of spinal column, through the tail bone and ending just above the floor surface, evenly spaced between your two feet.

Overview of Your Posture Indicators

Now you have some well documented information about differences between each side of your body. These are your indicators for planning future muscle training body movements.

Self-Assessment at its Best

You may be wondering about the painful areas that did not show up in this assessment. Possibly, the uncompromising Three Tenets are reminding you to look into regions where your body harbors "hot spots" and their *hidden agenda*. Discomfort coming from these "hot spots" indicates an area under strain. They are mostly found by applying pressure. Some will not be news to you, others a surprise; some will linger for some time, while others will disappear during your therapy sessions.

A variety of tools are available to help you detect these areas. Some practitioners use varying sizes of balls, rollers and other circular objects designed for muscle manipulation. I found them very effective when they were accompanied with directions from qualified

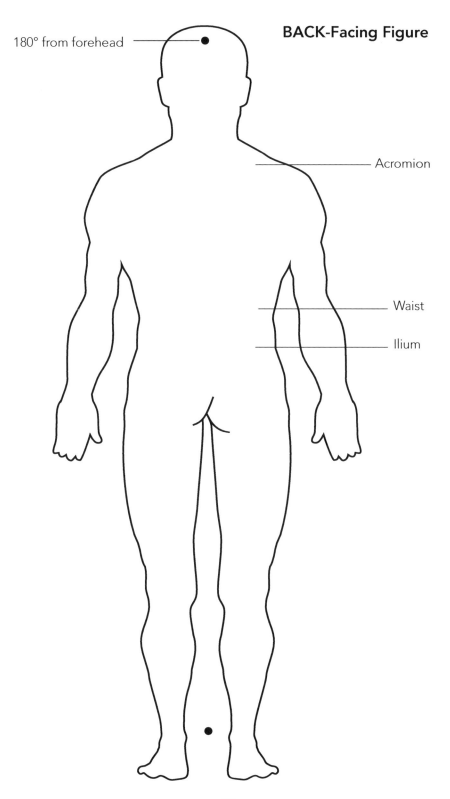

180° from forehead

BACK-Facing Figure

Acromion

Waist

Ilium

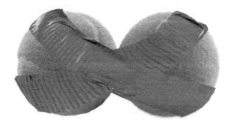

health professionals. My favorites are a roller called Power Point Roller, and four tennis balls bundled in twos (put into a sock or taped together). I can roll on them, placing them under various body parts to locate areas responding to the pressure, thus in need of further manipulation. Do not work with these pressure-finding tools without learning more about using them properly.

Directions for locating "hot spots" and *hidden agenda* should meet the standards put forth in this book in order to adequately fulfill your expectations

More information on these topics is developed in more detail in the chapters following. Chapter Four introduces elements of change for making choices, thus decisions, about treating your physiological and biological structure. Chapter Five written by Dr. John "Ed" Fellow, explains the effects imbalances have on our musculoskeletal system. Before making your selections from the body movements in Chapter Fifteen, you will learn about scientific theories and practices that will prepare you for getting control of your thoughts and developing your strategies for managing your musculoskeletal system. Some of your accomplishments will be enhancing motor memory and cognitive skills, and coming into close contact with your interior body design, while accepting the architectural responsibility for its form and function.

Using Your Information

Having completed both self-assessments has given you improved understanding of your body structure. You have just answered the first question, *Do I have some skeletal muscles in need of repair?* In so doing, you are closer to answering the other two: *If I do have misalignments, how bad is the condition?* and *How can I fix them?* Without further hesitation, direct your energy toward making use of the scope and sequence of the contents presented in each of the remaining chapters.

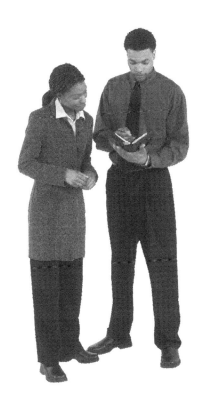

4

GAINING PROPER PERSPECTIVE

CONCEPTS FOR CHANGE AT WORK WITH *VIS VITAE*

The Squared Away approach includes having a descent process for making changes. These Concepts for Change are not complicated and are easily used as guidelines for making changes in your life, not just in body structures. As you use these Concepts to interpret what you discovered from making the self-assessments, you will find them to be both compatible and creditable conventions for making choices.

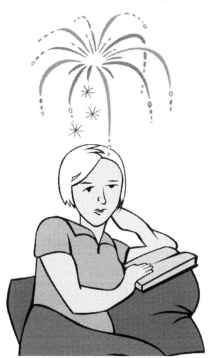

So, before you decide on the changes required to meet your physiological fitness criteria, give some consideration to your desires, and select one or two you would like to accomplish during the years ahead when enriching your physical fitness aptitude and lifestyle. These goals are called *vis vitae*. They are referred to throughout the text.

***Vis Vitae* Become Your Destiny**

Your *vis vitae* will become forces in your life—they are vital sparks on which you can concentrate your energy along with your knowledge and thoughts. Your responsibility is to begin thinking about a few physical attributes that are exceptionally important to you, important enough to be called "forces in your life" or *vis vitae*. Making the decision to keep these elements active will elevate your potential for successfully achieving and maintaining a neutrally structured—**Squared Away**—body alignment.

Concepts for Change

Titles of the six Concepts for Change describe their purpose. Clarifications of each title appear opposite the bullets; sometimes cross-referenced in the text so you can connect them with subjects being discussed. Hopefully, as you read through the chapters, you can relate all six Concepts and begin using them throughout your life.

Concept #1 *Misalignments* Disrupt Form and Function

- The Three Tenets guide our thinking about misalignments and keep us focused

- Answering the Three Questions keeps us directed

- Myofascial and neurofascial networks make connections among bone, muscles and other body tissue

- Misalignments occur when our posture is abnormal

- Many of us have problems with muscle performance.

These concepts on *misalignments* are covered in Chapters One through Nine and Chapter Thirteen. They help us to locate and improve poor muscle performance.

Concept #2 *Positive Direction* Comes from Knowledge

- The brain controls our contact with the world

- Our skeletal muscles are controlled by the brain

- Reconfiguring our musculoskeletal system begins with self-awareness

- Our thoughts guide our muscle performance

- Our force-of-life selections, *vis vitae*, help us to find and sustain muscle efficiency and effectiveness

- **Thinking, remembering, awareness, analysis and application** can lead to motor memory (also known as motor learning)

Information about **Positive Directions** to use for achieving better alignment and muscle mechanics is covered every chapter.

Concept #3 *Quality Attracts Attention*

- The Squared Away Principles are guidelines for acquiring a straight and even body structure
- There are attractive attributes to having a straight and even body structure
- Good posture promotes good performance
- Pilates has a special dialect deserving our full attention

Chapters One, Two, Three, Four, Six, Nine and Ten explain how to include *Quality* in our everyday activities.

Concept #4 *Physical Fitness Has an Attitude*

- Research has given us knowledge of past scientific accomplishments
- Physical fitness has many interpretations
- Physiological fitness refers to the neutral structure of human anatomy
- This book also defines physical fitness as being the same as being Squared Away—being physiologically fit or Having Our Act Together
- Realizing the inroads that physical fitness has made in our lives, gives us insight

Emphases on having an *Attitude*, on physical fitness and on the definitions of terms are made mostly in Chapters Five, Seven, Eight, Nine and Ten.

Concept #5 *Success Breeds Confidence.*

- We need to take responsibility for our body condition

- Self-actualizing Skills refer to: Self-awareness Skills, Self-assessment Skills and Self-management Skills

- Paying attention to our senses, especially visual and touch, in order to visualize and feel proper muscle movement, quickens our achieving a neutral anatomical body structure as well as motor memory

- Anatomical planes of motion and basic directions of muscle movement are important concepts for us to understand

- Pilates Breathing and Stance Principles are fundamental to correctly practicing body movement exercises

- Pilates Principles can be an adjunct to other physical activities we enjoy.

These concepts — *About Success* — are developed primarily in: "You First", "Breathing Principles", as well as in Chapters Two, Three, Five, Six, Seven and Nine.

Concept #6 The Squared Away Body is Universally Appealing

- When appropriately disciplined, muscles establish natural posture

- Performance deserves intelligent attention

- We look better when we feel better

- The Squared Away body structure is a neutrally anatomical body structure

- Having our Act Together is a worthy destination

- We need a long-range plan and lots of patience to keep us focused

Every chapter offers knowledge leading to confidence in having a *Universally Appealing* body and developing skills for restructing and improving our muscle appearance and function.

Concepts For Change Go To Work

These Concepts were designed for you, the problem-solver. They are the "trial-and-error" survivors of many guidelines attempted when deciding which were essential to evaluating progress toward reaching our *vis vitae.* Here is an example of how to proceed.

Suppose one of your **vis vitae**, is to eliminate chronic pain in muscles located in and around your left scapula. Look at the Concepts for Change # 1, #5 and #6. Each has qualifying statements about the pervasive nature of misalignments and the value of having long-range goals *(vis vitae)* as well as recognizing the Three Tenets.

Concept #1 *Misalignments Disrupt Form and Function,* introduces the concept—because of misalignments, our body does not perform nor function correctly. The statements opposite the bullets help us focus on ways to improve our physiological condition.

- The first bullet refers to the three questions also mentioned in Chapter One. They remain with us, helping us to answer the **Three Questions**: *Do I have misalignments? How bad is the condition? and How can I fix it?*

- Once we have answered the first question, the second bullet refers us to the **Three Tenets**. The First Tenet suggests that misalignments can go unnoticed, consequently going unattended. Therefore, it is not unusual to experience imbalances in our body structure.

By making use of the **#5 Concept for Change,** *Success Breeds Confidence*, the statements opposite the bullets provide us with additional details for interpreting our self-assessment discoveries.

- Putting to work what we know about using our kinesthetic skills, Self-activating Skills and Breathing Principles help us treat areas needing improvement.

Concept for Change #6, *The Squared Away Body is Universally Appealing*, tells us that the Squared Away body alignment creates a healthy, interesting and well structured form and function.

- Such attributes deserve intelligent attention. Being in control of our Whole Body Health offers opportunities for sustaining and improving our skeletal body condition.

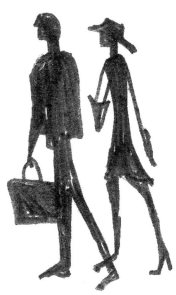

Making Application

Learning to be discerning becomes a major component for gaining control of your physical efficiency and effectiveness. Spend some time to select one or two *vis vitae* and write them in the space below.

Vis Vitae

_____

_____

Select the Concepts for Change that will be most helpful to you as you work to accomplish your *vis vitae* which have become sparks in your life, worthy of lasting pursuit. More information on reaching these objectives is in the following chapters.

5

IMBALANCES NEED DIRECTION

Doctor John "Ed" Fellow completed his family medicine residency degree at the University of California at San Diego, where he served as chief resident. He spent several years in private and group practices in both Family and Sports Medicine. In 1998, he joined Scripps Clinic and today practices non-surgical orthopedic sports medicine, with an emphasis on treating musculoskeletal injuries. Dr. Fellow is currently practicing at Scripps Clinic, Rancho Bernardo, in San Diego, California.

Reflections

Through twenty-five years of practicing sports medicine, I have found that practicing medicine is indeed an art form. My contacts with thousands of athletes and not-so-athletic patients every year have shown the results and value in matching treatments that correct a variety of dysfunctional skeletal conditions. I have been very fortunate to be a staff member at Scripps Clinic, practicing Orthopedic Sports Medicine. Being associated with exceptional physicians, therapists and other colleagues throughout the Scripps organization has widened my appreciation of the many forces that are intricately involved in healing. Solving puzzling problems and resolving patients' medical issues provide immense rewards and a tremendous sense of self-worth. There is nothing like having contacts and experiences, both personal and professional, to rely on when trying to tell someone what to do, what *not* to do and what to do next.

Collaborating with Mary and writing about how misalignments relate to the Squared Away principles has been a pleasure. Mary has taken great strides bringing the past to the present, while presenting to you a worthy approach for shaping a healthier Whole Body future. By using these principles, with diligence, you will find success in developing skills for establishing a ready, relaxed and centered body posture. Perhaps, in the process, you will discover the best performance-enhancer.

As you recall, for the purpose of this manuscript, we have taken the liberty of interchanging the terms, "imbalance" and "misalignment", when referring to the same irregular conditions in skeletal muscle form and function. I am using the term, imbalance, in this chapter to incorporate both form and function to describe *atypical* postural conditions in the human body. Along with using preventive treatment and improvement procedures, Squared Away concepts—at all times—consider the Whole Body Health even when recognizing that body posture is a primary indicator of body alignment. Therapists locate atypical tissue and muscular irregularities by tracing the origin of pain and postural alignments. Therefore, body posture is considered to be a major indicator, identifying deviations in the musculoskeletal system, not visa versa. The bottom line is that poor posture causes poor muscle performance. Squared Away takes these principles, measures them and essentially finely tunes them.

Cause and Effect Relationships

Regardless of how the postural discrepancies occur, there are some similar symptoms among imbalances that give signals to their location, and the severity of their intensity. I mention these "like-conditions" because during your self-assessment, you were asked to find imbalances using pressure technology, with tennis balls and other pressure identifying practices. This brings up the more noticeable characteristic — pain.

The "hidden agenda" imbedded in areas that are sensitive to pressure are reliable indicators of muscle imbalances, and should not be overlooked. Although the pain may not be severe at first, they are important signals needing attention. Let us examine some examples of cause and effect relationships.

Most imbalances are accompanied by various degrees of pain or discomfort, thus causing a domino-effect as they progress through various stages. First, when skeletal muscles experience extra stress, weakness follows, which then leads to failure in the supporting tissues, bones and cells of the musculoskeletal system. These failures challenge the body's coping skills, subsequently over-loading it by putting pressure and strain on normal muscle function. Without having proper diagnosis and feedback taking place, early in the cause and effect cycle of misalignments, critical communication, organization and treatments are delayed or lost.

Starting at the centers of pain, and extending via the domino-effect into other parts of the body, a generalized breakdown occurs when congestion and commotion take over. Such disabilities limit the body's ability to begin repairs. Of course, as another domino falls, this can lead to thick stacking or scarring, which becomes difficult to repair.

Did you know that within the next half-century, nine out of ten Americans will be suffering from back pain at sometime during their lifetime? Furthermore, eight of the nine will have recurrences of these pains. It is important to notice that these statistics do not even include problems associated with neck and other skeletal muscles, or joint problems. No wonder doctors are so busy.

How do these *atypical* body conditions occur? If they do, what is the treatment for them? What can be done to prevent them from happening to you? These are the questions you want to be asking at this point in your learning-curve.

Remember in the first few chapters when you were introduced to the Squared Away approach and given information on using the Squared Away principles to "Get your Act Together?" Well, this problem-solving process also requires having reliable and sufficient information to help establish practices that measure-up to those included in the medically sound and Squared Away recommendations. You can count on these practices and this information to meet the highest standards imposed by professional technicians and physicians. Reliable resources are grounded in sound science and application procedures.

Misalignments and their Direct and Indirect Effects on Body Performance

Every day our body encounters numerous physiological obstacles that can add to, or detract from, our musculoskeletal efficiency and effectiveness. Imbalances disrupt the Whole Body Health; whether *directly* or *indirectly* impacting the system—sometimes this is referred to as the "one-thing-leads-to-another" or "contagion," syndrome.

When imbalances *directly* affect the skeletal body structure, there is weakness, not only in the affected areas, but throughout the body. Pain is rather intense at first, builds with time and possibly subsides in a few weeks. Immediate pain or any pain that comes soon after the invasion of our muscles can actually help in the diagnoses by isolating dramatic findings responsible for increased misery. They often are more concentrated and can be quickly treated if occurring abruptly from specific injury types. Some examples would be: (1) collarbone or clavicle fractures (2) most ankle fractures (3) tearing of tendons such as Achilles or biceps. Also, these direct invasions are less likely to be the origin of widespread damage.

Indirect effects from imbalances are more sinister, causing small effects that eventually show widespread damage. Because their point of origin is quite subtle, possibly less shocking at first, they are difficult to trace and follow. These characteristics can cause the patient to massage his/her shoulder when the area needing treatment is in the neck or spine. Another misinterpretation can come when the patient has persistent indigestion or an upset stomach. If the cause is from physiological imbalance, tension increases neurotransmitters which, in the case of serotonin, can affect body mobility, hormonal and gastrointestinal balance. Such hormonal changes are not good companions to your friendly body structures. They can distort our sense of balance and contribute to further discomfort, stress or insomnia. The entire neighborhood can become an irritable disorder.

Misalignments that Occur Abruptly and Cumulatively (Overtime)

In Chapter One, you were reminded that muscular imbalances can take months and years to be noticed; these are designated as being *cumulative* misalignments. On the other hand, when imbalances occur *abruptly*, the opposite timeline is responsible for the disruption. Either way, imbalances occur because the muscles are unnaturally positioned, thus performing unnaturally. As you might imagine, when our muscles experience an *abrupt* invasion without time to prepare for it, such disruptions can be very damaging. However, when imbalances occur cumulatively, they can be equally, if not more, damaging to our Whole Body Health. If the skeletal muscle and surrounding tissue have been mal-functioning for long periods of time, an unnatural and rigid mass can become quite a problem. Reconditioning such deviations can take years.

Misalignments from: Under-using, Over-using or Mis-using Skeletal Muscles

Misalignments from Under-using Our Muscles

Daily, I see patients with skeletal muscle **"use problems"** due to: misusing, over-using and under-using their skeletal muscles. These are skeletal muscles or imbalances that have "gone amuck."

Body Systems

Cardiovascular and Circulatory—blood circulation, heart, blood and vessels

Endocrine—communicates with body hormones

Excretory—eliminates body waste

Immune System—defender against disease

Integumentary—skin, hair and nails

Lymphatic—network of vessels that transports nutrients and waste

Muscular—moves the body with muscles

Nervous—interacts with the brain

Reproductive—sex organs

Respiratory—nose, trachea and lungs

Sensory—includes ears, eyes, nose, skin and tongue

Skeletal—structural support and protection through bones

With the **under-use** of our skeletal muscles and tissue, they become ineffective, mainly due to dehydration and stiffness which reduces their stamina and performance.

Because the human body is two-thirds water, a very delicate balance exists in order to maintain a healthy Whole Body balance. Each system in our body (see Box) runs on water.

These systems are intrinsically interdependent as they manage the distribution and collection of body liquids. Therefore, any disturbance can disrupt the interdependency between this delicate flow and balance. The outcome is an inappropriate increase in hydraulic pressures and disorderly rhythms; therefore, the changes in pressure, both physically and chemically, cause pain and subsequent breakdowns in the body's systems. Thus, raising havoc throughout the twelve body systems, especially damaging and lowering the body's immune system. The alert defenses are compromised and invaders and cell terrorists get implanted.

Personally Speaking

You can appreciate the value of drinking water before, during and after any physical activity, i.e., exercising or playing sports. I tell my patients to, …"first drink water, water, water—then drink sports drinks and add a little salt too." They also hear other quotations like, "Disease has a harder time Catching you when you are on the Move, and are Well-hydrated and In Balance." Another favorite is telling them, if they slow down their pace of practice and participation, their perspective about the important things in life can be better appreciated. The idea is to practice better for greater play, staying relaxed, but ready to "make it happen."

Misalignments from Over-using our Muscles

Over-using our muscles can be equally damaging because instead of just causing excessive hydration or dehydration, the level of muscle tolerance is being abused. Many of the breaks or stress fractures that I see and treat are the result of *not* applying the *brakes* soon enough. Not having enough regularly scheduled breaks or rests result in distress. We fall victim to not including cross-training and balanced practices. Sometimes we just keep going at the cost of experiencing permanent injury and delaying normal growth patterns. I am particularly heartened when I can help young adults and children, early in their lives, to use new habits, chart a safer course by staying more patient and slowing down so they can focus and enhance their every day life.

Misalignments from Misusing our Muscles

Misusing our skeletal muscles is an on-going event that happens frequently because we are neglecting our Self-activating Skills. The number of occasions in which these disruptions can occur is huge.

Misuse of Muscles and Self-Activating Skills

We have found that daily practicing Self-activating Skills is an essential component of preventive medicine. You will also find them contagious. Once you start looking at your own body analytically, you begin noticing the postural condition of everyone else. Such behaviors are excellent habits to have.

Personally Speaking

Recognizing that improving, maintaining and *specializing* our muscular integrity is a lot of work; it can also be a lot of fun. Finding ways to laugh, even at ourselves, is good medicine for all of us, especially those who are intense sports competitors. I encourage my patients to spy (I.S.S.P.I.) because this generates relaxed practicing of Self-activating Skills while improving muscular integrity. The athlete is trained to *specialize* in using her/his: Intellectual, Spiritual, Social, Physical and Intimate realms (I.S.S.P.I.).

Athletes Are Unique

Although you and I are not quite as intense as the athlete, in moderation, we still need to follow the same methods and techniques when rejuvenating and renewing our skeletal muscles. The athlete and non-athlete both have goals he/she wants to accomplish to master their *vis vitae*. They just use varying degrees of intensity and focus.

As an athlete, you in particular, like to know that your advisors are proficient in your particular sport, and have first-hand understanding of the dynamics involved in playing sports such as: being a team member, acknowledging that the whole is greater than the parts, and learning how to handle success or injuries that can affect one's psyche, etc.

I hope you are keeping a personal log to track what goes on during your practices: the minutes spent in certain actions, evaluating your practice and jotting down muscle movements on which you need to focus during your next workout, and/or think about, in the interim. In other words, are your timelines being met? Are your practices structured to include specifications for: (a) hours of rest and sleep (b) specifications for diet (c) attitude adjustments (d) putting to work your Self-activating Skills (e) continuing instructions on achieving a Squared Away body condition and performance? The ordinary person and the athletic performers need to monitor wisely the hours and the calibre of demands made on their muscles in any given performance or practice. I know that my patients are best served when prescribed activities include reasonable restrictions.

Staying ready, well postured and neutrally positioned keep all of us moving and feeling well.

Encouragement to You, the Reader

So, whether you are trying to find procedures for making repairs that will *improve, maintain* and/or *specialize* your physical body condition, do not forget the impact that repeating correctly, repetitive movements, have on making these adjustments. Recreation or sport participation is all about rejuvenating and renewal. How many hours has this dancer spent on acquiring such a beautiful pose? I know for a fact that the many muscles at work here are in her motor memory bank. They have been deposited daily over many years. Meet my daughter Jessica Fellow.

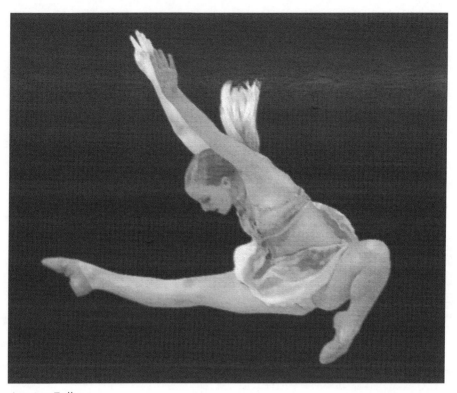

Jessica Fellow

Staying patient and steadfast helps everyone prepare for success. Take time out to recall the advantages of having a repertoire of extensive motor memory, as it is paramount to keeping your body moving automatically. One begins by (a) consciously performing, over time, repetitions of specific muscles, then (b) adding associated kinesthetic awareness of those movements and ultimately (c) they can become completely subconscious and part of his/her motor memory.

Mary has brought together, through this book, unlikely companions to explain the Squared Away concept. She has given the reader exposure to external—worldly influences—that can be internalized and personally embraced to enrich our lives. By digging deeper and mastering these principles, you can achieve your *vis vitae*. As you share your experience with others, the circle becomes complete.

6

SCIENTISTS AT WORK

Facing Reality

This chapter spans events that have taken place in past and present times. It brings into focus some of mankind's progress toward meeting expectations for obtaining a healthy and well-aligned body structure. The chapter explains the: (1) control that the brain has over muscle performance, (2) the composition and performance of skeletal muscles and (3) application of skills learned, and knowledge gained, for making improvements in the body posture and condition.

Staying Patient

Before becoming "master" of our physiological destiny, we need to know all we can about the characteristics of our skeletal muscles that can affect their performance. The last half of this book addresses these topics, covering some of the distinctive features of skeletal muscle performance and structure. Augmenting such areas of study are suggestions for maintaining these acquisitions as they become life-long attributes for establishing and sustaining a youthful, stable, strong and reliable body form and function.

You have taken time to discover some valuable information about your body posture and performance by making your self-assessments and learning about the importance of making changes

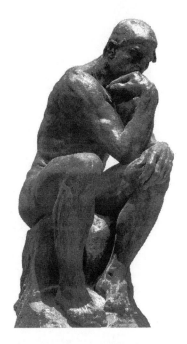

Rodin: The Thinker

in your muscle composition. You may be anxious to get-on with the project and go directly to the chapter titled, "Body Movements Take Shape", so you can start working with some exercises. Some other approaches to becoming physiologically fit might suggest such hasty transitions. However, the Squared Away approach emphasizes being well-informed and personally involved before attempting to use any body movement practices. Learning about the ancients is one of these precursors.

Whether *improving*, *maintaining* or *specializing* skeletal muscle, you are participating in a lifetime excursion that is best taken in progressive steps of difficulty. Gradually, reading each chapter reduces errors as you select levels of body movements to practice and set the pace at which you practice them. The Squared Away method makes a point of preparing you to act independently, knowingly and with confidence. After all, you are building a structure that will be timeless. Possessing certain knowledge of the ancients is a good place to begin. It gives us reference.

Starting with the Ancients, 460 B.C.–201 A.D.

They made it happen! It has been over 2400 years since the Greeks began studying human anatomy. They began looking at the likes of you and me, attempting to understand — the structure of human beings, and wanting to know — how this inner composition was

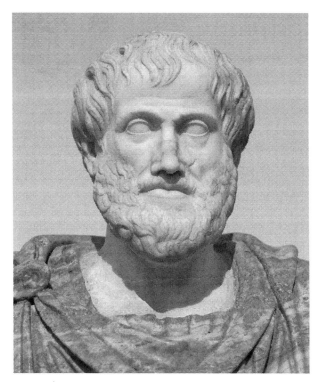
Aristotle

linked to their thoughts, minds and brains. The work they conducted
and procedures they followed would set high standards for future
studies and scientific perceptions about muscle function and their
interactions with the human brain.

Quite typical of those with inquisitive minds, finding agreement
on interpreting their discoveries can *not* be easily obtained. A Greek
physician, Hippocrates (460–377 B.C) concluded that the mind was
in the brain and controlled by the body. Plato, a philosopher and
mathematician, born in 427 B.C, agreed with Hippocrates that the
mind was in the head, but specified that the mind and body were
separate. Aristotle (384–322 B.C) the Greek philosopher, biologist
and thinker wrote on many subjects. He was a student of Plato and
a teacher of Alexander the Great. His opinions on physical sciences,
specifically on the mind-brain issue, were that the mind and brain
were one.

It was much later that a Roman physician and philosopher,
Claudius Galen (131–201 AD) described muscle structure and
function, believing muscles were contracted by "swelling", a

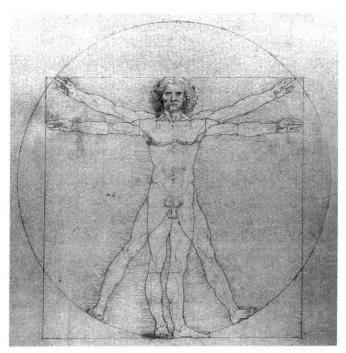
The Vitruvian Man by Leonardo da Vinci

movement determined to be inherent. He proposed that the body was kept alive by forces residing in the brain, heart and liver.

In later years, opinions were voiced by others who would argue support of, or disagreement with, theories about the "mind-body connection." Through the ages, impressive proposals have continued to stimulate investigations of these connections.

Others Who Made a Difference 1400–1600 A.D.

During the middle ages, research in anatomy and physiology was quite sparse. Not until the sixteenth and seventeenth centuries, would research in human anatomy be revisited with consistency. A great deal has been written about the Renaissance of Muscle Research that began around the 1500s. In these times, understanding human anatomy, biology and physiology were also made by notables other than the scientist.

Prominent artist drawings would add to theories being proposed by those conducting scientific research. Andrea Vesalius (1514–1564) an artist, anatomist, physician and writer, composed one of the more influential books on human anatomy. This book titled, *On the Fabric of the Human Body*, contained his drawings showing locations of muscles in the human body. Andrea's work is still a resource to artists, students and scientists. Likewise, Leonardo da Vinci (1452–1519) and Michelangelo (1475–1564) had a thorough understanding of anatomy and mastery of form and movement giving their artistic creations remarkable accuracy.

These artists had "hands-on" exposure to the human body structure. Such practical experiences with the human musculoskeletal system greatly influenced their superior and singularly magnificent works of art.

Personally Speaking

I have made a modest selection of geniuses, mentioning a few among many, who made remarkable contributions to our enlightened understanding of these complicated topics. My intention in offering you this slight glimpse into the past was to call your attention to a few studies that were conducted so many years ago. At the same time, I wanted to insure recognition of how arduously our ancestors over the last two thousand-plus-years applied themselves to such discoveries. If they had not, I am not sure at what level today you and I could be discussing the Squared Away body structure. As we move on, yet still holding onto our thoughts about these early studies, we begin to look at more modern times—the last half of the twentieth century.

Moving Ahead When Misconceptions Abound 1950–1980

While others began taking advantage of these advancements, some of us were not staying current with the progress being made. My friends and I were still disciplining our body structures for efficiency and strength. It would take some years before we realized that the Squared Away body was *not* a body described as being well-disciplined, somewhat rigid and possibly misaligned.

Flexibility and balance were not mentioned as often as were tactics for disciplining muscles for performance. One can look great in stretch jeans and form-fitting tops, but without flexibility, one's body movements can look horribly awkward when performing everyday musculoskeletal movements.

During these years, joggers who ran on concrete and asphalt surfaces were formidable obstacles-in-motion to the pedestrians who with them negotiated these narrow sidewalks. Some of these creatures, while presenting a rather iconic image while streaking through neighborhoods, would later suffer from having ground-up cartilage in their vertebra and knees, fallen arches or sagging jaw lines. I'm not making fun of these sports men and women. I was one of them, never iconic, but often one of the obstacles-in-motion, and sometimes interfering with my fellow pedestrians — pressing onward, harder and harder.

Adding to this scenario, both sexes under the guidance of their coaches, instructors, physical therapists, trainers, etc., were taking advantage of the myriad of "physical fitness" offerings. Branches from physiological, biological and anatomical sciences that investigated theories on muscle dynamics, were becoming increasingly important to those instructing muscle movement and body performance. Such influences were included by enlightened professionals who designed physical therapy and physical fitness activities. Not only the athlete, but the ordinary citizen, was benefiting from discoveries taking place in biomechanics, geometry of movement, neurological and electrophysiological technology, to name just a few.

Stepping into the 21st Century, Facing Up to Reality

How are you getting along with balancing the many roles you have in your life — parent, caregiver, student, worker, sports person, homemaker, etc.? Is your body holding-up under the strain? Can you easily eyeball your putt on the putting green or with agility get out of a car or look over your shoulder without having to turn your upper body to do so? The more desirable response would sound something like — "Yes, I can, and with a neutral anatomical (normal) body posture."

If, for even one day, you are able to make all of these movements without compromising your neutral anatomical body posture, you have a day to remember. For the rest of us, by using our pressure tactics such as rolling on tennis balls or rollers, we will find tranquility by massaging our muscles and improving our musculoskeletal system using appropriate body movement practices.

Maybe you are aware that you, like many others, have spinal deviations or a persistent region of pain in your body. Seldom are the topics of posture, alignment or back and neck irritations brought up, without people talking about having similar pain and inconveniences related to these unpleasant conditions. Of course, feeling sorry for ourselves and complaining about our health problems, will not solve our problem(s). Hopefully, no one will try to resolve the situation by removing all the mirrors in the house. I found relief when listening to the wording in a song written by Jimmy Buffet—*Margaritaville*—, words that rang true to me when the lyrics repeated...."*it's my own d— fault.*" After I accepted responsibility for: possibly self-inflicting, and certainly, for self-sustaining my alignment problems, half of my battle was won. Ownership was not as challenging as I feared it might be.

Chapter Seven gives you a chance take a breather and relax a bit.

7

A COMMON LANGUAGE PREVAILS

Unintentional confusion occurs rather easily if the reader is unsure of the author's wording. We can avoid such misunderstandings by reviewing a few definitions typical of what I call the Squared Away "speak." This is a "clear-the-air-list" of some words and terms that will lighten your read through the remaining chapters.

Let Us Define Terms

I thought you would welcome a change of pace while digesting content covered in the first chapters. The Squared Away approach has no intention of leaving you stranded and without assistance to find your way through the most important and difficult phases of body alignment processes. Having a common language between us gives us an even playing field as we tackle out-of-the-ordinary topics.

Definition of Terms

These definitions are slanted toward how they have been used in the context of this book.

Aponeurosis is a sheet of pearly-white fibrous tissue that takes the place of a tendon when the muscle has a sheet-like region needing attachment to bone. It serves as fascia, binding muscles together for connecting muscle to bone.

Fascia is a thin sheath of fibrous tissue enclosing a muscle or another organ.

Fitness is the condition of being physically fit and healthy.

Kinesthesia is the sensation in the body of the movement of muscles. (*Webster's College Dictionary*). This harmonious association is said to exist between the brain and muscle contractions—making muscle movement possible.

Motor Memory (muscle memory) takes place when the muscle repeatedly moves in a specific pattern. When combined with our senses, our ability to repeat specific muscle movements transcends our conscious efforts, and becomes part of our motor memory repertoire.

Muscular endurance is a health-related fitness component that relates to the amount of external force which a muscle can exert over an extended period of time—without fatigue.

Muscle Form and Function refers to the physiological and anatomical properties of our own body structure.

Muscle Strength and Efficiency are mentioned together in the text because they are integrated partners when developing a neutral anatomical body structure. When properly specified, they even-out our body form and function—making possible a well-aligned and natural physical performance.

Myofascial pertains to the fascia surrounding and separating muscle tissue. Now commonly considered to be synonomous with soft tissue.

Neurofascia refers to a network of nerve cells and fascia that extends throughout the body.

Physical is used when referring to the body, as opposed to the mind.

Physical Fitness is the ability of the body to respond or adapt to the demands and stress of physical effort.

Physiological means the branch of biology that deals with the normal functions of living organisms and their parts. The way in which a living organism or bodily part functions, i.e., the physiology of the brain.

Physiotherapy a British term for physical therapy.

Whole Body Health means being psychologically, anatomically and physiologically fit.

Expansion of Terms Using Squared Away "Speak"

Sometimes terms or some grouping of words, are confused with one another, in the pages following, are some clarifications for your

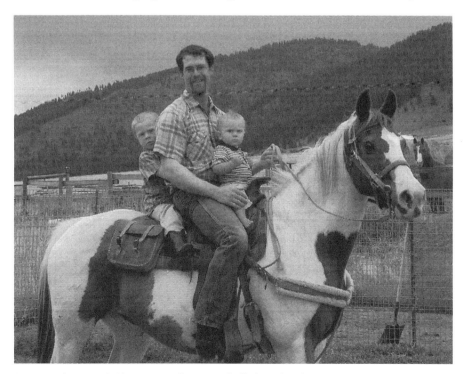

Case, Tobin, and Clayton make use of all their body parts.

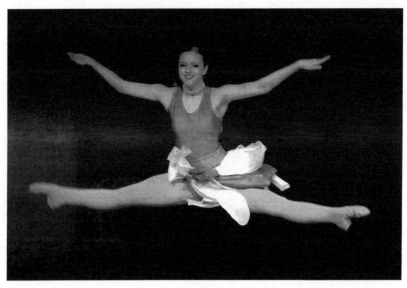

Jessica

consideration. **Physiological fitness** and **physical fitness** deserve top priority because they are often misinterpreted.

Physiological fitness describes the condition of the structure or the parts of human anatomy.

On the other hand, there seems to be no silver-tongued definition of the term **physical fitness**. Have you noticed how frequently **physical fitness** is used when lumping together an inordinate number of body-related topics? Many sources ask us to indulge in certain foods, beverages, dietary products, various practices and activities, programs etc. — all referring to being physically fit. Sometimes entrepreneurs promote physical fitness products claiming them to be change-agents for making us physically attractive, youthful and healthy while improving our memory, too. Such generality creates a problem because providers have their own interpretation of physical fitness and, unless defined, we can only guess at their intentions.

For the purpose of this manuscript, I have narrowed the term "physical fitness" so you know what I am writing about when I use it. Physical fitness is defined as a body structure possessing the Squared Away body structure—unencumbered and ready to move in balance with natural flexibility and strength.

In other words, using the criteria in Squared Away Self-Assessments, you are describing a body in which each side of the body is within ½ inch of its partner. Also, the string when free-falling reveals the same dimensions when measured between body points.

These two terms: **kinesthesia** and **motor memory** are often connected because they have a strong cause-and-effect relationship. When consciously activated, both voluntary and involuntary muscles are responsible for movement of our body. As we work to normalize some body movements, and are consciously thinking about the feelings associated with these special muscle movements, such attention—with time—can develop motor memory. Kinesthesia becomes highly affective under these circumstances. However, we should not be misguided in thinking that such changes are regularly possible. Unusual discipline is required.

The terms, **muscle strength** and **efficiency** have been used to describe an obedient and well-structured body, getting high grades for being efficient. Muscle strength has taken on an entirely different meaning—it is no longer confined to describing power or muscle building. Physiotherapists, along with other professionals in the fields of health, helped those of us wanting a more flexible body condition—less rigid, yet strong without looking muscular. Along with the idea of training muscles to meet different outcomes, muscle strength and efficiency were linked together, but with less emphasis on strength and more on flexibility.

Today, you can recognize practical application of this approach by seeing it included in many physical disciplines that emphasize both muscle form and function. Many instructors of yoga and Pilates, plus certified physical therapists, along with those in medical fields, specialize in using an anatomical and physiological basis in their instruction and corrective measures.

Whole Body Health always seems to need clarification. It is used in this text as a reminder that being physiologically and mentally fit, includes being constantly in contact with:

■ our *Self-activating Skills* — which keep us practicing self-awareness, self-assessment, self-management and

■ our thought processes, so we are daily applying the valid information as we move through our everyday life style, and accomplishing our *vis vitae*.

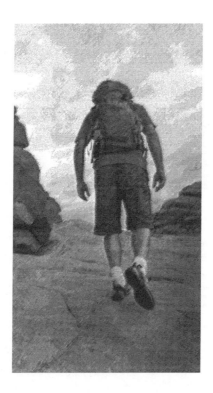

8

OUR BRAIN TAKES CHARGE

OUR THOUGHTS MANAGE OUR ACTIONS

Appreciating our Partnership

When I began writing Squared Away, a top priority was to insure that the content was organized so you and I would have a compatible working relationship. I wanted you to be comfortable accepting the information I would be sharing with you. Together, we would convert it into authentic and practical physiological activities, as well as establish thought management sequences to meet your individual needs.

You have certainly been a good sport—responding in preceding chapters to some unusual requests for your participation. Consequently, between the two of us, your body condition has transcended guesswork, and you are making steady progress toward realizing your chosen *vis vitae*.

Scientific support behind the Squared Away principles, when combined with your knowledge and insights on the subject, are an excellent footing for investigating the role the brain plays in putting into motion the musculoskeletal system. A natural extension of such understanding is to condition your muscles so that their movement can be repeated either consciously (on-call) or through motor memory (unconsciously). When making such movements and concentrating on them, the sensory feeling compliments the

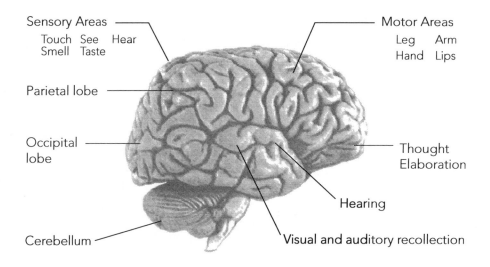

Sensory Areas
  Touch See Hear
  Smell Taste

Parietal lobe

Occipital lobe

Cerebellum

Motor Areas
  Leg   Arm
  Hand Lips

Thought Elaboration

Hearing

Visual and auditory recollection

activity. As you recall, combining one's focus with desired repetitions of muscle movement, enhances opportunity for installing what is commonly referred to as motor memory. Let us discover more about the functions of the brain so you can take advantage of its cognitive possibilities.

The Brain Is in Charge

Our brain is in control of coordinating a whole range of conscious (voluntary) and subconscious (involuntary) muscle activities. It is known for being the most complex system in the human body. Whenever we have both practical knowledge and reliable interpretations of facts concerning how our brain controls muscle movements, we are well-equipped to *improve, maintain* and *specialize* or (embellish) our skeletal muscle performance.

    Often, senior citizens are quite curious about relationships between physical exercise and the impact it has on mental capabilities. Actually, this is a good question for all ages. You may have similar thoughts about the effects that our physical and mental stimulation have on keeping the brain alert. Information in this chapter exposes some of the discussion involved in connecting physical activity with cognitive function and cognitive aging.

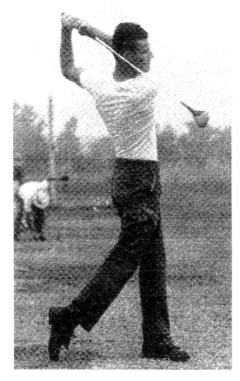

Barry McDonnell

Gaining Perspective of the Whole Person

Kinesthesia, which is described in Chapter Five and Seven, deserves our attention here because of the brain's activity involving the sensation that detects the position, movement and tension of our body parts. Simply defined, such stimuli are the result of interactions between the brain and muscle movements. We have recognized the impact felt within our body structure when muscle training is combined with conscious intention. Kinesthesia, when joined with our conscious thoughts over time, can result in motor memory. Content in this chapter explains this connection.

Questions and Answers

Examples of motor memory, are those muscle movements that are performed automatically and repeatedly, such as: using the keys of a keyboard, riding a bicycle, using tools or eating utensils, driving a car, playing a musical instrument, etc. By increasing the number of motor memory items that you have stored away, you can spend more time paying conscious attention to muscle movements in need of active thought management. What voluntary muscle movements would you like to add to your memory bank?

When we think about performing certain muscle movements while moving them, opportunity for installing motor memory is enhanced.

> Would an efficient use of your time be to expand motor memory so that some muscles in your musculoskeletal system could perform without your conscious efforts? Would you say that being focused by paying thoughtful attention—when repeated over time—could make it happen? How would you do that?

_____

_____

Research Worthy of Your Time

In the left and right hemispheres of the brain there is a very small curved structure called the **hippocampus**. Among other responsibilities, the two hippocampi are involved in consolidating information from short-term memory to long-term memory. Normal aging is often associated with gradual loss of memory. Some studies reported shrinkage in the brain of elderly people, while others have not produced such findings. Research continues investigating the relationship between aging and memory loss. Declines in memory are often apparent before the occurrence of other problems in memory such as dementias, and can cause reduction in cognitive ability such as Alzheimer's disease.

Consensus has been gathering, stating that aerobic exercise can promote chemical change in the hippocampus. These changes directly affect the brain by increasing the brain protein, called BDNF (Brain-derived Neurotrophic Factor) which acts as a "fertilizer," nourishing new connections between neurons. This factor has an infinity for certain nerve cells or tissue, and selectively localizes them.

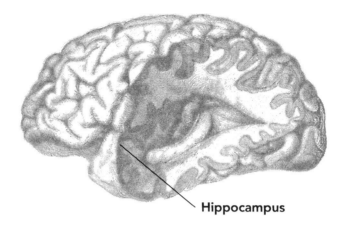

Hippocampus

Over the past decade, progress has been made in determining effects that aerobics fitness training has had on cognitive function and brain health. The first study of its kind—that focused on older adults who were already experiencing atrophy of the hippocampus—was conducted by researchers from the University of Pittsburgh and the University of Illinois, Rice University and the Ohio State University. Findings of the study have been published in several health magazines and research documents such as: "*The Archives of Neurology*" (Vol. 67, No. 1) and in the "*Proceedings of the National Academy of Sciences*", January 2007, also referenced in the Bibliography.

Aerobic Exercise and Cognitive Memory

Doctors, Arthur Kramer, director of the Beckman Institute at the University of Illinois at Urbana-Champaign, and Dr. Kirk Erickson, professor of psychology at the University of Pittsburg, were the senior and lead authors respectively, of the project. Dr. Kramer said during a National Public Radio interview on February 21, 2011, "What we found is that individuals in the aerobic group showed increases in the volume of their hippocampus." Dr. Erickson wrote in the report of findings…"we think the atrophy of the hippocampus in later life as almost inevitable." He went on to say they had shown that …"vigorous activities stimulate the heart and increase oxygen consumption are beneficial beyond cardiovascular health." Exercises used by the participants included: fast biking, fast walking, jogging, or running.

Currently, other studies are being conducted to investigate **neurogenesis (**the creation of new neurons) especially in the **hippocampus**. Within these investigations, interesting data have surfaced about the production of compounds, sometimes called "fertilizers", that energize both synapse and neuron production. Staying current on progress being made in these scientific examinations of the brain and of human cognitive skills, can guide you when making choices about enhancing your brain health.

Conclusions

It appears that by increasing brain flexibility — which means changing its structure and function — we can enhance responses we make to input being received. And, here is the "kicker!" Such changes that occur when responding to input, are strongly affected by *attention*, which can alter brain physiology and enlarge its functional circuits. You can stay well-informed on these topics, and keep learning more about them, by reading publications covering Whole Body Health.

I can *not* think of a more significant outcome from this discussion than to put into practice what we have learned about staying focused or being attentive. The concept highlights the importance of staying focused, using our Self-Activating Skills for being successful.

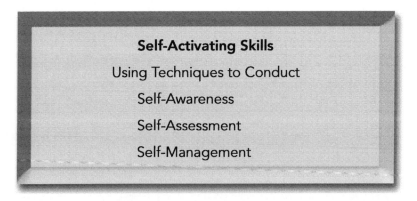

Self-Activating Skills

Using Techniques to Conduct

Self-Awareness

Self-Assessment

Self-Management

We are cautioned about trying to accomplish cognitive enhancement strategies until more information is available. This is another example of how undefined terms can suggest products and practices to accomplish unreliable goals.

An article written by Sharon Begley, with Ian Yarett, "*Newsweek Magazine*", January 10 & 17, 2001, identifies a neuroscientist from Columbia University, Yaakov Stern. Dr. Stern gives credit to greater cognitive capacity coming from creating more neurons (neurogenesis), especially in the **hippocampus**, along with increased levels of compounds that can lead to neurogenesis. His findings have led to concluding that such increases in the neurogenesis process can stimulate production of neurons and synapses.

Mentioned in the article are random studies that cite various practices and products to make us smarter. It seems that training in specific tasks can improve ability in the task being taught, but does not generalize to others. However, it is encouraging to note that the brain can be modified, and that one year of moderate exercise by those in this age group could *reverse* shrinkage of the hippocampus.

Personally Speaking

It is appropriate to mention here that some people with respected credentials have challenged the validity of these findings. Yet, I found little substance to their criticisms. I have concluded that those over age sixty with, the right amount and type of aerobic exercise, when coupled with **attending** to the kinetic properties of the muscles

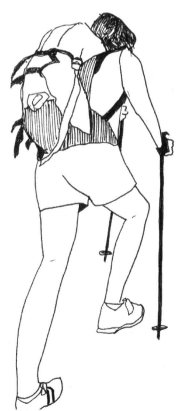

being trained, can increase opportunities for improving memory, reasoning and creativity.

What are your conclusions or has your experience been inconclusive? Possibly, you will take note regarding your cognitive performance after following a regimen of aerobic exercise similar to the one used in the Beckman Institue study. I would appreciate hearing from you regarding this activity.

Getting Your Mind around Thought Management

We have just reviewed statements about realizing benefits gained by paying **attention** to the dynamics taking place as our mind and body structures interact. Thought management follows a natural sequence, calling for us to use our brain to **think, remember** and **be aware** of the task at hand. As we apply our thoughts and analyze outcomes, the cycle is completed. In other words, constantly analyzing our techniques, to guide and perfect our performance.

It is never too early or too late to adopt this sequence.

Ponder this picture. I wonder what sport each of these girls will try. Who knows what can happen? It looks like they may have some trouble finding an indoor court on which to practice tennis, but they could follow Picabo Street, Olympic Gold Medalist, and tackle the slopes. They could even receive an Olympic Gold.

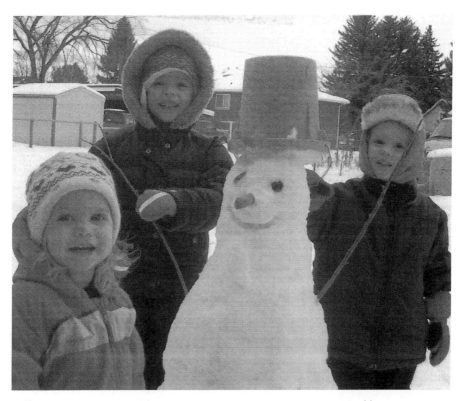

Tiffany   Haley   Madilynn

9

SKELETAL MUSCLES KNOW THEIR PLACE

Taking Charge of Self-Management

> During your life, you have brought together your knowledge and skills in order to get things done. The journey that you are making in reading this book shows that you are inspired about taking intelligent care of your physical condition. Having the confidence to make changes in your body structure is truly a wonderful accomplishment.

Here we are in Chapter Nine and you are being asked to inspect your muscular composition, and the structural support of it, in order to manifest a flexible, energetic and aesthetic body condition. We will be looking at the interactive characteristics of the forces within our body structure that make movement possible. Action taking place throughout the musculoskeletal system depends on the combined effort given, and the character created by, bone, tendons, tissue and ligaments. Of equal importance is the calibre of the mental and cellular intercommunications activating these structures.

Recalling the attempts that were made over the past two thousand-plus-years by those trying to understand how energy takes

Posterior View

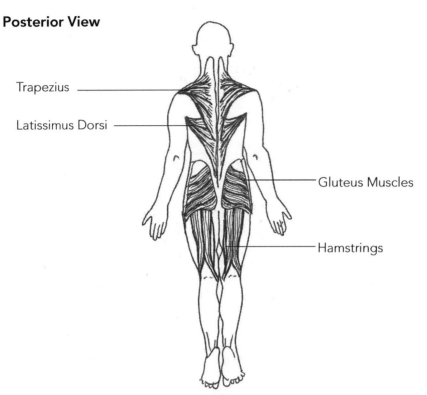

Trapezius

Latissimus Dorsi

Gluteus Muscles

Hamstrings

Anterior View

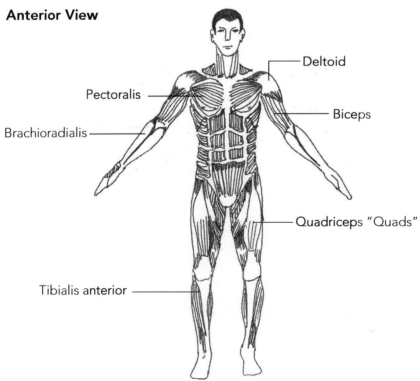

Deltoid

Pectoralis

Biceps

Brachioradialis

Quadriceps "Quads"

Tibialis anterior

place within the body structure has a way of keeping us humble. We take for granted today what has been for centuries in the making. Particularly when discussing the efficient and effective dynamics of trillions of cells simultaneously contributing to movement of a finger or toe, by generating electricity to energize such muscle movements. We can now use these findings to help us manage their performance.

Bones, Connective Tissue and Muscles

Although there are basic components of the human body, there is great opportunity for variety to exist within our individual body structures. Each human body is unique in so many ways because of the varied shapes and types of bones, joints, connective tissue and muscles that comprise the musculoskeletal system. This chapter investigates these common, yet individual, interconnections affecting our body's flexibility, or restrictions of it, as we move about during our daily activities.

You will be privy to professional insights that were thought through, with YOU in mind. Information centers on investigating your muscle composition and function so you can control these aspects of your life as you realize your life's visions or *vis vitae*.

Self-managing your musculoskeletal condition becomes increasingly more accurate when you have knowledge about the skeletal muscle levels of force and endurance. This information is paramount when deciding how to treat your musculoskeletal condition, and taking the appropriate steps in order to *improve*, then *stabilize*, unnatural posture when it occurs. Such sensitivity has special relevance when choosing the body movement exercises to make the necessary changes.

Muscle Types: Heart, Smooth and Skeletal

Movement taking place in our body structure depends on contraction of our muscles. Structures of muscles found in the human body fit into three main categories:

Types of Human Muscles

Heart (Cardiac) Smooth and Skeletal Muscles

Smooth and Cardiac muscles are called involuntary because movement is mostly automatic and occurs *without* our consciously initiating it.

Skeletal muscle is called voluntary because these muscles move *with* our conscious intention.

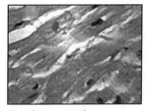
Cardiac muscle

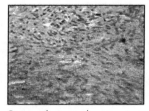
Smooth muscle

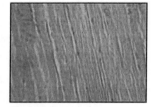
Skeletal muscle

Heart (cardiac muscle) is found only near the heart. Smooth muscle is found in the walls of blood vessels, the digestive tract, and in the skin where microscopic bands of muscle connect hair follicles to the skin (called the arrector pili).

Characteristics of Skeletal Muscle

Because the content of Squared Away deals mostly with our physiological and anatomical body form and function, the rest of this chapter covers the skeletal muscle category.

Skeletal muscles comprise the largest number of muscles in the human body, over 640, and account for around 40 percent of the body's mass. They are primarily controlled by the nervous system, activated by our thoughts, and also have the ability to move powerfully and quickly. These muscles are recognized by a striated or striped appearance.

Skeletal muscles are composed of fibers which are bundled together by fibrous partitions described below. These fibrous partitions, by forming layers of fibrous tissue between and among the fibers, have different levels of packaging. Although continuous with one another, each level has special properties for making connections possible.

Fibrous Partitions of Skeletal Muscles

Epimysium is a thin, yet fibrous and elastic tissue that wraps a muscle.

Perimysium fragile layer inside the muscle, surrounding individual muscle fibers.

Endomysium is a thin and delicate connective tissue surrounding individual muscle fiber.

Perichondrium, covers cartilage (except at the joints) enabling muscles to connect to cartilage.

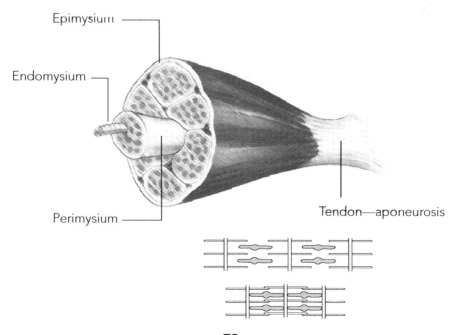

Epimysium

Endomysium

Perimysium

Tendon—aponeurosis

Our skeletal muscles are composed of two kinds of fibers: **fast twitch** and **slow twitch**, which produce different levels of muscle contractions. Quite frequently, the example used to explain the **fast-twitch** and the **slow-twitch**, compares the sprinter to the marathon runner. The **fast-twitch** generates short bursts of speed as contrasted to the **slow-twitch**. The more sustaining **slow twitch muscle fibers** generate a rather low-level of force output, yet resist fatigue for longer periods of time. This chart is an easy reference for this information.

Types of Skeletal Muscle Fibers

Type I produces slow-twitch contractions, needed for long-lasting endurance to fatigue

Type II refers to fast-twitch contractions, they have a low-level tolerance for fatigue

Type IIa can hold a steady pace and be fairly resistant to fatigue

Type IIb generates more power and force at faster speeds than any other fiber

Musculoskeletal Characteristics and Dynamics

By staying connected with information, and being informed about how muscle movement occurs, we can avoid putting too much strain or unknowingly mistreating our skeletal muscles. You have just read about their composition and potential for creating various levels of movement. Another significant consideration for *improving*, *maintaining* and/or *specializing* our muscle performance would be considering how our muscles attach to bone. With a few exceptions, movement in our body takes place by muscle contractions that are orchestrated by muscle attachments to bone.

Muscle points-of-attachment to bone or other tissue have a give-and-take relationship. Because our muscles have different connections to bone, and occasionally to other tissue—as in the mouth and face—these various attachments highly influence muscle performance. Knowing more about these connections enables us to use intelligent judgment when moving them; therefore, avoiding strains, misalignments, etc. It IS true that good information precedes good performance.

Avoiding muscle and/or tendon strain is a matter of using good judgment to protect your musculoskeletal system from unusual stress and intervention. Since our body posture and composition are considered to be a process-in-motion, muscular conditions are always in flux. Yet, accidents can be minimized, and certainly can be avoided, when we consciously use our Self-activating Skills to observe and take proper action when improving and/or maintaining a neutral anatomical body structure. Such persistent conduct has the potential for becoming life-long assets, and with habitual repetitions, they can even become motor memory. What behaviors are you working on that you would like to see "motorized" or performing, involuntarily? You can make your decisions about being connected as we progress.

Staying *Connected* with Tendons, Ligaments and Cartilage

Tendons, ligaments and cartilage connect muscles to body tissue.

The **Tendon** is a dense fibrous tissue or cord that *connects* muscle to bone. It has different shapes—some have flat layers with a sheet-like appearance (aponeorosis) and others are dense with a more flexible fibrous tissue. Often, tendons are referred to as: the strongest substances in the body, capable of withstanding injury as in ruptured muscles and broken bones. They are part of the neuromuscular system; and electrical charges flow through them in order to reach muscle tissue. It is wise to give a little TLC to these "work horses" and make their burdens less intense.

Ligaments are said to be arranged in parallel bundles. They appear, resembling an elastic band or sheet of tough fibrous tissue that *connects* bone-to-bone, bone-to-cartilage in the joint areas, and bone-to-bone when supporting an organ. Their main function is to act as stabilizers and to strengthen joints. With the exception of a few instances, they do not contract.

Cartilage covers articulating surfaces of bones with a shiny whitish tissue. This *connection* protects underlying bone tissue.

Staying *Connected* By Origin and Insertion

Over the last 30-40 years, studies that were conducted on muscle attachment or *connection*, often used the terms origin and insertion. Muscle *points* of attachment are designated as origin, and insertion is located at the *ends* of the muscles. Generally, a muscle is attached to two bones. The point of attachment, where the muscle is fixed in position, is called origin. The point of attachment to a more movable bone is called insertion. Another way of looking at body movement is to recognize that it is an interaction of muscles contracting across joints.

Staying *Connected* With Purpose

Recent researchers are still looking for answers to similar questions that the ancients were trying to answer. The quest for discovering the sources responsible for moving the human body has been a challenge for thousands of years. Throughout the centuries, scientists have shown little reserve in dismantling an unassuming, comatose partner when trying to solve this illusive mystery. Unraveling the elite and singularly-formed function and structural composition of the human body remains an occupying force for many who are recognized for

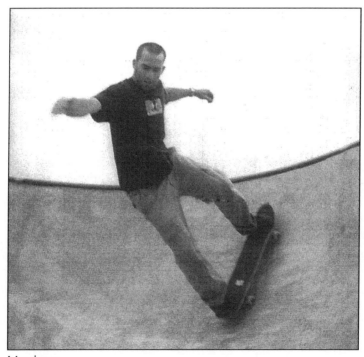

Matthew

their great intellect and persevering purpose. On a much smaller scale, you are engaged in the same pursuit as you self-manage your physicality—investigating and *connecting* proven principles of your musculoskeletal system.

Staying *Connected* With Electrical Properties

Another influential area shedding light on how our muscles move, involves knowing about electrolytes. Where exactly does the energy come from that is responsible for causing our muscles to move? Modern science tells us that the human body is composed of emerging fields. And, in order to have optimal performance, there needs to be a steady *connection* supplying the nutrients being carried by the electrolytes.

The molecular nature of electrolytes has chemicals which have the ability to conduct electricity thus, helping mankind to maintain proper energy levels throughout the body. Electrolytes are chemical substances that are electrically charged; therefore, producing electrically charged particles (ions) in our body fluids. These ions keep the cells healthy by supplying sodium, potassium, bicarbonate and chloride. Cells use this salt compound to govern metabolism, conduct impulses along nerve fibers and to regulate muscular contractions. Changes in the chemical concentrations in and around our nerves, produce an electrical current which can move our body. Although, such action is much more complicated than this simple explanation, basically, our nerve cells are responsible for our body movement, while our brain manages performance.

The ancients wanted answers about how the body moves. Who would have thought that muscle movements take place by generating electricity to energize them? Today, you and I can use these findings to help us manage our body condition. We can look directly at remote connections of our musculoskeletal system.

Possibly you will begin taking more precautions than you have previously taken to protect your body's efficiency and effectiveness. "Looking at the Real You" in Chapter Ten will help you personalize the information you have gained from reading and participating in activities presented in the first nine chapters.

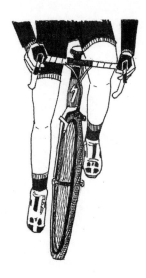

10

LOOKING AT THE REAL YOU

Muscles Have Huge Responsibilities

In the last chapter, you reviewed the characteristics and dynamics of how our skeletal muscle, tissue and bone perform so that movement of this musculoskeletal system is possible. You have a good understanding of how a neutral anatomical body structure should be connected, what it should look like, and how misalignments have a penchant for disrupting our body's normal form and function. As you read this sampling of illustrations and descriptions of various tissue → to → bone connections, take time to visualize and associate them with your own skeletal muscle connections.

For those readers who have a background in using technical terms to describe human muscle performance and composition, please be patient with the explanations that I have used when describing these topics.

Muscle Attachments to Bone: Direct and Indirect

Explanation of Direct Attachment

A few skeletal muscles attach directly to bone via muscle fibers at their insertion and origin. For this reason, they are described as having direct attachments. Here is one example — located in our upper torso.

Direct Attachment

SHOULDER-ARM

Posterior View of Subscapularis

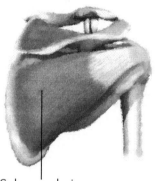

Subscapularis

Muscle Description and Location

The subscapularis is just what you would expect, the muscle fibers attach directly or are attenuated (the muscle fibers become flat, concave and fringed at the origin and insertion). This is a large triangular muscle that helps connect the arm to the shoulder. The muscle fibers originate from the scapula and insert on the humerus. It is one of the four muscles forming the rotator cuff.

Subscapularis: Normal Muscle Performance

When performing naturally, and other muscles in the area are working together, the movement would include rotation, elevation and depression, abduction and adduction. Collectively, they mobilize the long arm bone (humerus) and guide the movement of the joint. The muscle plays a major role in stabilizing shoulder irregularities

Treatment

Consider using body movement exercises that help with flexibility, strength (not rigid) and alignment of the neck and shoulders; also including those associated with the vertebrae and upper torso muscles. Taking care of our shoulders and arms is more than a pastime. These muscles can benefit tremendously from your practicing the Pilates Breathing Principles, thus keeping the shoulders neutrally positioned.

Indirect Muscle Attachments to Bone

Explanation

Most muscles fit into the indirect attachment category; in fact, most of the bones in our legs and arms qualify. A muscle is said to be indirectly attached (sometimes called the fleshy attachment) when the muscle ends before the point on the bone where the muscle should attach. This gap between muscle and bone is filled by a tendon.

These muscles have origin in bone and are inserted to bone at another connection by different-shaped tendons. Because tendons have a more fibrous nature than the fleshy texture of muscles, the majority of skeletal muscle connections are made by tendons. On the next pages are examples of indirect connections from different parts of our musculoskeletal system.

SHOULDER and NECK

Anterior View of Deltoid

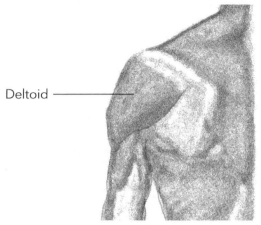

Deltoid

Muscle Description and Location

The deltoid muscle forms the rounded contour of the shoulder. An illustration of the deltoid muscle (commonly called the shoulder muscle) gives a clear picture of an indirect attachment. It consists of three groups of fibers that attach to the acromion, scapula and the surfaces of the humerus. These fiber groups enclose the middle surface and insert on the outward (lateral) surface of the long arm bone or humerus.

Deltoid: Normal Muscle Performance

The deltoid contracts these three fiber groups on the front of the muscle and performs flexion and medial (frontal) rotation of the arm.

Treatment

Body movement practices using these muscles would include those that internally and externally rotate the shoulder. Keeping these muscles flexible in the entire shoulder area will help with neck and shoulder flexibility.

NECK and BACK

Posterior View of Levator Scapula

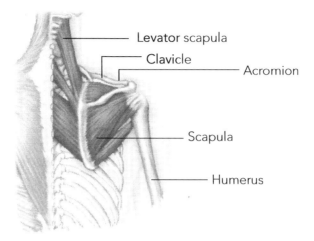

Levator scapula

Clavicle

Acromion

Scapula

Humerus

Muscle Description and Location

These muscles are located on each side of the neck and insert along the inside scapular borders. They originate from a bone projection on either side of the vertebrae, called the transverse process, and insert along each scapula, inside the border that is (superior) or toward the head.

Levator Scapulae: Normal Muscle Performance

Work with your neck and shoulder muscles while using your self-assessment to guide your movements. As the human head moves, around 600 times in one hour, you can see the value of maintaining a flexible and Squared Away head and shoulder alignment—thus posture—with flexibility.

ARM and ELBOW

Anterior View of the Brachioradialis

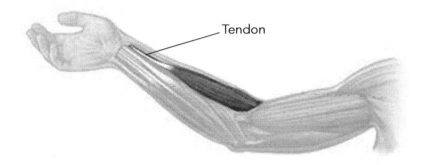

Tendon

Muscle Description and Location

The brachioradialis originates from the outer (lateral) ridge of our upper arm long bone (humerus) and inserts just above the wrist. This muscle has direct attachment to the outer edge of the upper arm bone just above the elbow, and inserts at the tendon on the same side, just above the wrist.

Normal Performance and Treatment: Brachioradialis

The major function is flexion of the elbow. The lower part of the arm (forearm) can be rotated toward or away from our center line. Use self-assessment information to select the body movements to move these body parts. Stretching, bending and straightening your arms, along with other shoulder practices are good body movements to include in your regimen.

HIP and KNEE

Anterior View Quadriceps Femoris

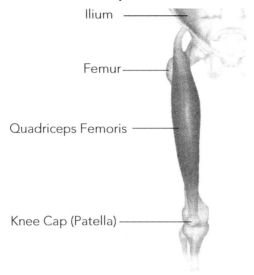

Ilium

Femur

Quadriceps Femoris

Knee Cap (Patella)

Muscle Description and Location

I chose the massive muscle, quadriceps femoris, as an example because we are constantly contracting these leg muscles as we support the rest of our body. This large muscle has three other muscles that function together in the upper part of the leg. They form into one tendon that inserts and surrounds the knee cap (patella) and finally forms a large tendon that inserts into the large lower leg bone (tibia).

Normal Quadriceps Femoris Muscle Performance

Most of the body movements made by this muscle group extend and rotate the knee and surrounding body parts. In some ways, almost every body movement exercise involves the movement of these muscles.

Muscle Treatment

It is almost impossible to isolate movements involving just the hip or knee. So, when selecting your body movements and practicing them, use discretion about how much energy is appropriate for your body condition. Body movements that lengthen the leg muscles and bend the knee are good stabilizers. Chapter Fifteen has quite a few for you to consider.

FOOT and ANKLE

Anterior View of Tibialis Anterior

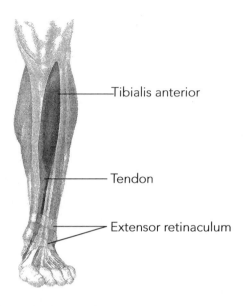

Tibialis anterior

Tendon

Extensor retinaculum

Muscle Description and Location

Some muscles take unusual routes from their origin as they pass over and under tissue and bone before insertion. The tibialis anterior is an example that is easily recognized because it is used in many instances to describe the front of the leg and foot. The illustration shows you the lengthy journey this muscle takes as it extends down the side of our leg and passes under the extensor retinaculum, finally inserting on the base of the big toe bone, hallucis.

Normal Muscle Performance and Treatment: Tibialis Anterior

The tibialis anterior is the strongest muscle that lifts the medial edge of the foot. It is involved with every step you take as well as other knee and ankle movements. Body movements in Chapter Fifteen that illustrate how to care for ankles and feet—they should be part of your regimen. Flexiblity and endurance are maintained with massage, plus leg and foot extension and rotation exercises. Walking and standing correctly are also important.

Insuring Progress in Your Physiological and Biological Form and Function

As you practice your body movement exercises, you can take advantage of what you know about the different ways in which our muscles attach to bone. Pulled or strained muscles can be avoided when you give special consideration (TLC) to these sensitive areas, especially when stretching and putting unusual strain on your bone-muscle connections.

Such caution is particularly advised whenever you are bending and flexing your legs and arms. This **antagonistic pairing** becomes a team effort as one muscle is bending while the other straightens. Such coordination takes continuous nutrients and balanced stamina as the **agonist** produces the movement, and the **antagonist** relaxes and produces the opposite action. Also, be aware that recent research has been focusing on the elastic properties of tendons and how they function as springs, indicating that tendons can also modify forces of movement within the musculoskeletal system.

Looking Ahead

Having learned more than you thought you wanted to know about skeletal muscles, we can move on to the chapters ahead and complete the cycle of establishing a Self-activating life style with maximum independence to make intelligent choices. Managing your thoughts and memory, self-awareness and a sense of feeling will help you analyze what it takes to establish an energetic and distinctively persuasive relationship with your inner body.

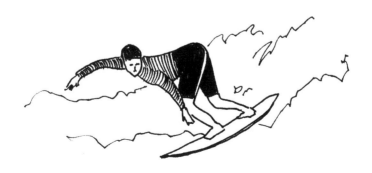

11

TAKING A BREATHER, STANDING TALL

WALKING with CONTROL

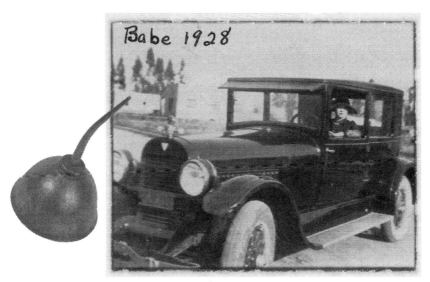

Frances—my mother

Are you ready for a breath of fresh air while you walk and stand? Learning to breathe properly is fundamental to Whole Body Health, and standing tall makes it possible. Carrying these principles forward and using them as you walk and stand, will be quite energizing to you, and genuinely attractive to others. Participating in Whole Health practices will help you to strengthen, lengthen and gain control of your body movements. Joseph Pilates and W.J. Miller describe these three principles in *Pilates' Return to Life Through Contrology*.

Managing Our Breaths of Life

Breathing correctly makes all movement seamless, especially when exercising and moving from one exercise to another. Standing tall will give you distinction and allow your breathing to be more effective. When combining these two practices and walking with control, you are well prepared for most of your skeletal body movements. As we move about during our day, our postural alignment will be attractive to others and reassuring to you because you are strengthening, lengthening and gaining control of your body movements.

Joseph Pilates emphasized proper breathing and standing in order to enhance body control. You can compare your ability to breathe correctly with the function that the oilcan had when lubricating the moveable parts on the early automobiles. Likewise, when we take air *deeply* into our lungs, we are lubricating our entire body and keeping our body moving smoothly and reducing long-term wear.

Joseph Pilates defined *"Contrology"* as a science that helps us lengthen, strengthen and control our body. As we gain control, we are able to transfer our muscle performance to all aspects of our musculoskeletal body movements.

Since I am not writing a book on anatomy, descriptions and directions are brief by comparison, yet helpful if taken slowly.

Breathing correctly involves timing, coordination and strengthening of specific respiratory muscles. Classic Pilates breathing suggests breathing through the nose and exhaling from the mouth. Pilates directions refer to using our powerhouse, which is considered to be the workhorse of the Pilates method, to stabilize the process. The powerhouse is comprised of the abdominal and the lower back muscles, as well as those in the hips and buttocks.

As you practice this brief interpretation of Pilates Principles of Breathing, be sure to avoid raising your shoulders or pushing your abdominal wall outward as you inhale. If you lie down when following these steps, add to the exhaling process, using your abdominals to tilt your pelvis slightly upward.

- Empty as much air as possible from your lungs

- While keeping your powerhouse strong, inhale

- Pull your navel toward your spine by fully breathing into the sides and back of your ribcage

- You should be feeling your lower ribs expanding in all directions

- Slowly exhale so that you can make a hissing sound

- You will also want to feel your ribs pushing back against your back bone and

- Feeling your ribs coming together in front of and inside of your waistband

- Relax your ribs and lungs and begin process once again

- Install normal breathing by practicing whenever it is safe to do so; repetitions enable you to improve connections between your mind and body

- Think about muscle and structural positions that you want to make involuntary

- Pace yourself, remember Dr. Fellow's remarks about having "restrictions" in your regimen

- Stay patient, taking a breather should simultaneously be relaxing and constructive

- Remain flexible

Standing Tall

We can use this brief outline of the Pilates Stance to get ourselves positioned correctly when working to match-up to the neutral anatomical body structure. In the beginning of the book, when I wrote about "You First," you were introduced to the meaning of a neutral anatomical body structure. Standing tall follows the criteria used in defining Squared Away and the Pilates Principles of Breathing. Chapter Fifteen has another interpretation for your consideration.

- Heels are together

- Your big toes should be separated from one another by about four fingers

- Legs are close enough together to resemble a zippered-effect, so that as little light as possible is seen between them

- Squeeze the muscles in your pelvic region

- Keeping your abdominals firmly rounded toward the back of your spine

- Hang arms loosely alongside the body

- Stretch top of head toward ceiling

- Your weight should be slightly more on the balls of your feet than on your heels

- Your shoulders are over your hips and the spine is assuming correct curvatures

Walking under Normal Conditions

Since it is impossible to see what we look like when walking (unless on video), here are few fundamentals that help you to maintain neutral anatomical body alignment.

- There is a sensation of rocking our feet as we put our heel down on the surface

- The rest of the foot follows as our

- Weight shifts and moves toward the toes and balls of the foot

- The 26 bones, 31 joints and 20 intrinsic muscles in the foot plus

- The ankle joint along with bones in the leg and the surrounding tissue in these regions

- Support our body as well as make possible our ability to walk, run, etc., that we expect when being upright and mobile

Walking in Unusual Conditions

- When walking up a hill, continue using normal foot and leg movements

Sometimes when climbing a sloping hill grade, we slap the sole of our foot down on the surface. Moving our legs and feet in this manner can cause our knees to absorb the shocks from this foot placement.

Accommodate the up hill surface by bending your knee and rotating your foot as if on an even surface.

- When walking on other surfaces, use normal body posture and adjust your body to maintain a strong and flexible prowess. Most important is having proper equipment if climbing or hiking

If the surface is irregular, be cautious about where you put your foot.

- Much has been written to describe how to hold your muscles during each body movement. The flow between movements can become an aerobic experience. Pilates instructors can help you personalize this coordination

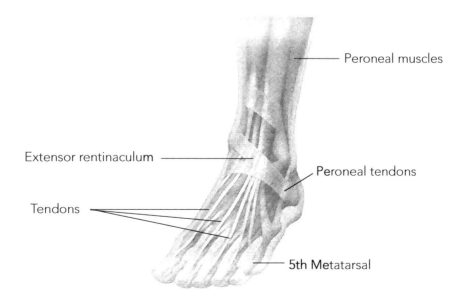

Peroneal muscles

Extensor rentinaculum

Peroneal tendons

Tendons

5th Metatarsal

Personally Speaking

For those of us who can move our bodies at will, sometimes we ask too much of our structural muscles. In all instances, we should show tolerance when training our muscles. This is a habit not easily developed, but of the utmost importance. Here is an incident pertinent to this statement.

Quite often I take walks on uneven paths, and carry a stick to ward-off wild critters that use the same trails. One day when beginning to learn the principles of breathing, I decided to practice them during my walk. At my stage of capability, this was not a good idea.

I was so busy cupping my hands around my ribs and trying to keep my feet correctly angled, that things went flying in every direction. The stick wasn't the first to hit the ground. Some people really learn the hard way. Before trying again to coordinate these activities, I went back to practicing in front of the mirror. With patience and time, I was able to develop a reliable kinesthetic relationship between the form and function of this mainstay for achieving proper postural alignment. Indeed, patience can be a virtue.

Many words have been used trying to explain and clarify the importance of, and process to use, when learning to breathe correctly. You can learn more about them from Cathleen Murakami who has written about classic Pilates methodology, chapter titled "Muscles into Action" in her book, *Morning Pilates Workout*. Of course, Joseph Pilates and William J. Miller recorded their original thoughts on the subject in their book *Pilates' Return to Life Through Contrology*.

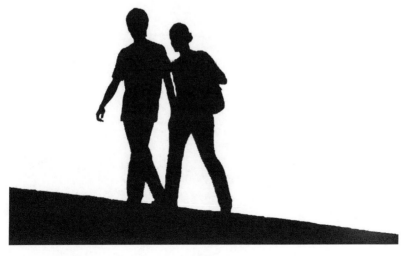

12

ANATOMICAL PLANES

BASIC DIRECTIONS OF MUSCLE MOVEMENT

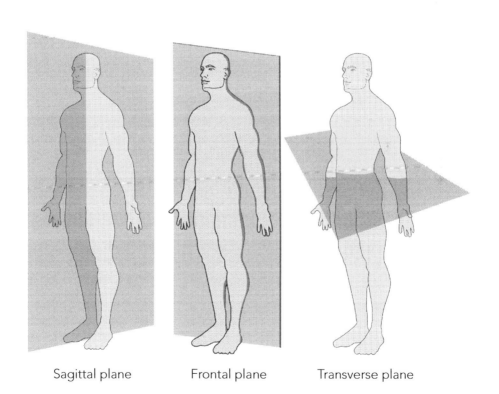

| Sagittal plane | Frontal plane | Transverse plane |

Directional Terms

In order to communicate with one another about the human body, directional terms have been developed by anatomists and physiologists to denote location and movements of our musculoskeletal system. These conventional terms use the *neutral anatomical position* as the point of reference. Throughout the text we have been in constant contact with this normal body condition. As you recall, the body is erect, eyes are straight ahead, feet almost together, toes pointing straight ahead, and arms at the sides with palms slightly forward and thumbs pointing forward — away from the body.

When referencing a given condition in your musculoskeletal system, having it described in general terms is not appropriate. You have probably heard about terrible incidents when the wrong body part was treated by a doctor. This chapter offers a means of using directional terms when identifying and sharing with others, specific locations and movements of your musculoskeletal system. You will be reducing lengthy language to describe anatomical, biological and physiological characteristics while increasing precision to explain and identify.

Anatomical Planes of Motion

Because our body structure is three-dimensional, there are three planes that slice through the body, dividing it into right-left segments, upper-lower parts and through the side of the body creating posterior (back or backward) and anterior (front or forward) sections.

The **median plane** divides the body *symmetrically* into halves, through the center of the body. Any plane that is parallel to it is called a **sagittal plane**. Body parts that are perpendicular to it refer to the **coronal** or **frontal plane**. The **transverse plane**, also called the **horizontal plane**, divides the body into superior (upper) and inferior (lower) portions.

Sagittal median

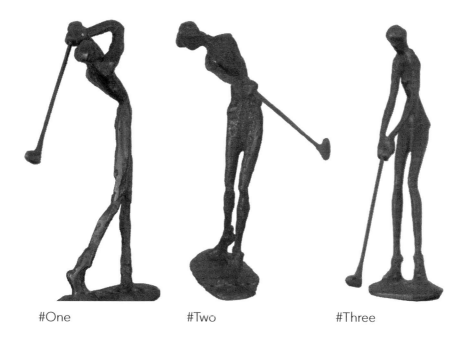

#One #Two #Three

Sagittal Plane

The sagittal plane is a vertical line paralleling the median plane and dividing the body into right and left halves. When referring to this plane, directions of movement describe parts of the body moving forward from an anatomical position such as raising an arm out in front of you. This is called flexion. Moving it behind you is called extension. One can easily see these movements when viewing the golfing figures #One and #Three from the side.

Performance

All three sculptures show how the golfer's arms and legs have moved forward and backward from the median plane. Before the swing is completed with the follow-through, the arms and legs will be flexing and extending twice on each side of the body. Shoulders, hips and knees are involved in executing these movements.

Coronal or Frontal Plane

The frontal or coronal plane is any line dividing the body into front (anterior) and back (posterior) segments; it separates the body through the side. The division is not intended to be symmetrical; it is applied arbitrarily by technicians to describe their particular reference points to anterior and posterior motion and location of the body parts.

Performance

Figure #Two shows the golfer crossing the right arm, wrists and hands in front of the body. When an appendage moves toward the median plane, the movement is called adduction. The left arm is moving more quickly away from the median plane, called abduction. Lateral flexion or side-bending takes place as the hands and feet have their own median plane; and the neck or trunk move away from the center line.

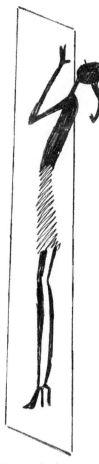

Coronal plane

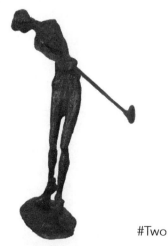

#Two

Body movements in
the coronal plane

Transverse Plane

This division fits any plane that is perpendicular to the median plane.

The transverse plane divides the body into top (superior) meaning situated above or directed upward, and inferior, describing body parts situated below or directed downward.

These movements are easily seen if looking down on, or up at, the body structure.

Performance

Movements made within this plane are said to be rotational. When a body part moves outward or away, it is making a lateral rotation (external); when the body moves inward, this is called medial rotation (internal). Movements can be seen in the legs as the backswing begins and the clubface is moving away from the ball. Figures #Two and #Three.

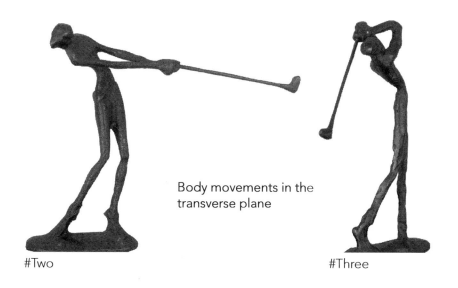

Body movements in the transverse plane

#Two   #Three

Displayed in the sculptures are other movements: supination, which is a forward or upward movement and pronation, downward or backward. Medial rotation of the shoulders is simultaneous as the golfer swings the golf club. When we are reminded why no two golf swings are alike, we can see why.

Definitions of Body Movement

For easy reference, here are the body movement terms used in the previous context.

Adduction - moves an appendage toward the midline

Abduction - moves an appendage away from the midline

Extension - moves a body part to the rear

Flexion - brings a body part forward

Lateral rotation - moves a body part outward

Medial rotation - moves a body part inward

Pronation - inward rotation of forearm causing palms to face downward, or foot to extend externally

Supination – outward rotation of forearm causing palm of the hand to face upward

This introduction is intended to help you observe and make comparisons of your body movements, noticing their ability to move forward, toward and above the center line, as well as back, away from and below. They can be a resource when monitoring your progress in flexibility, strength and range of motion that you noticed in your self-assessment and are now working to *improve, maintain* and or *specialize*. Whenever you feel the need for knowing more about these topics please consult the Bibliography for additional resources.

CHAPTER

13
DRAWING LINES FOR PERFECTION

Content in this chapter will move you one step closer to making a comfortable transition from simply looking at your body condition with indifference → to replenishing defective areas with functional and reliable muscle performance. You will be taking this information to the MAT!

Practicing Good Habits

Staying Alert

Do not be discouraged if you experience fluctuations in your muscle neutrality. It is not uncommon to have repetitions of an event like the one I mention next.

On Friday you can have full range of neutrally positioned muscles. Consequently, you decide to ignore your practice regimen over the weekend. By Monday, your body has so many "hot spots" you feel like you have been a target on a shooting range, although all you did was pull some weeds in the garden. And, further more, guess who is going to be responsible for fixing it?

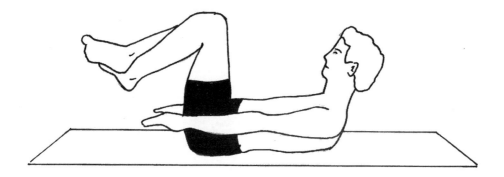

Sorry to report, but such events are not uncommon; they can occur weekly, and I mean weekly. This is just another reminder that our muscles are always "a-work-in-progress" constantly charting different configurations of movement requiring our attention.

Staying Patient

A positive attitude will make a difference in your progress. Self-awareness offers encouragement because most of us have muscles which are functioning unnaturally, and needing our attention. I have written about problems caused by postponing our search for reliable information. Experiencing persistent or intermittent pain and stress are early warning signals of trouble ahead. Dealing with them promptly, will be forever valuable when *fixing the problem.*

Redirecting muscles is labor-intensive and can also be frustrating and unrealistically prolonged. Realizing that these uninvited guests have taken their time to appear, helps us understand the time required in getting them realigned. We now have the unpleasant job of being an unaccommodating host until we can get them rehabilitated. That is precisely why we are spending this time together.

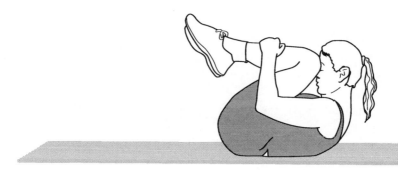

Your Practice Mat Becomes Your Partner

Constructing a practice mat might seem a bit pedantic or unnecessary to you. However, marking it is serious business. At no time in this text has more emphasis been given to being precise. Fundamental to achieving proper muscle movements is having a stabilized platform on which you have registered your body measurements. On this surface, while practicing your evenly-constituted formulae, you can replace undesirable alignments and ailments, with an evenly-proportioned posture.

Correctly scored, your mat becomes a reliable and trusted friend. It holds valuable guidelines for your quality control, reminding you that success depends on keeping the body on your Squared Away practice lines, while practicing thought management. By staying alert and improving your Self-activating Skills, Self-awareness and Self-assessment Skills, improvement in your musculoskeletal system is eminent.

Pre-activation for Marking Your Mat

Find a flat surface, large enough to accommodate your mat and still have room to walk around it. Place the material you are using on top of this surface. Your mat should be approximately 6–7 feet long, width about 26–35 inches. Have available several large safety pins and, if working with rubber or Styrofoam, you will need some Scotch-tape. You will also need: writing materials for record-keeping, a straight-edged marking object like a yard stick or measuring tape that can firmly hold its edge, and a water-proof marking pen.

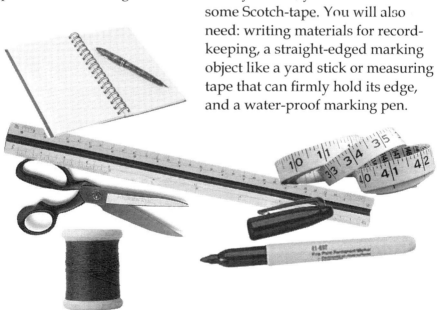

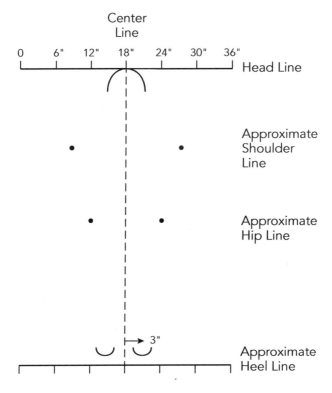

This project is more easily accomplished when you have someone to help you manage putting marks on the mat for your shoulder, hip and heel measurements. The illustration shows the markings you will be making on your mat to show your **head line**, **foot line** and **center line**, also your **heel**, **shoulder** and **hip lines**. Take time now to view your material as an overview.

Directions for Constructing Your Practice Mat

The material of which your mat is made should easily tolerate as well as retain, the lines drawn with your marking pen and the placement of your safety pins or Scotch-tape. Materials such as rubber or Styrofoam are often used. I used a queen-sized bed sheet folded in half. This was adequate when placed on top of carpeting. It also withstood many launderings. Because this material will contain all of your accurate measurements, vertically and horizontally, it needs to have well aligned margins.

1. Beginning at the left side 3–4 inches down from the evenly trimmed top of your mat, put a mark

every 6 inches across the top. Use a ruler to draw a horizontal line through these markings. This line is called your **head line**

2. To establish your **foot line**, measure down from **head line**, 6–8 feet, depending on your height. To form your **foot line** and have this rectangle perfectly aligned; begin at the same side as you did for the **head line**. Repeat measuring from **head line** down to bottom edge every 6 inches. Be sure the distances are evenly spaced on bottom line directly below the **head line** markings that were made every 6 inches across to form the line

3. Draw a horizontal line through these markings to form your **foot line**. Having these two lines accurately spaced is extremely important. *If there is a discrepancy, go back to the beginning and measure again so all points are perfect*

4. Measure the width of your material and divide number in half to mark the center of your mat

5. Draw a line down the center from **head line** to **foot line**; this is the **center line**

6. Put safety pins on intersection of **center line** and **head line**. If you are working with Styrofoam or plastic mats, use Scotch-tape

7. Lie down on the mat, back of your head is centered on the safety pins or Scotch-tape; spinal column is lying on top of the **center line**. Extend legs straight down below hips with heels evenly straddling the **center line**, 3–4 inches from it, and toes pointing toward the ceiling

8. Mark where your heels meet the mat surface. These two marks are your **heel lines**

9. Lying down once again, in same position, you will be using your **shoulder body points** that you made on the acromion (which is a projection on

the scapulae that forms the point on the shoulder and the collar bone). Do not readjust your body to place your shoulders evenly on the mat

10. Mark each side of your mat where your **shoulder body points** would meet the mat when you align a pencil from them pointing down to the practice mat

11. Draw a line on mat connecting these new markings; this is your **shoulder line**

12. Give yourself a dry-run while your "accomplice" is still available. Lie down on your mat and checkout all of the **line markings** with your **body point markings**. Fix those needing to be changed

On Target

Because you have been reading about the ancients, as well as others of scientific prowess, I am suggesting that you keep their accomplishments in mind as you take on the world, and show caution when preparing and practicing your body movement selections. Chapter Fourteen gives you an interview with an important character that you will not want to miss.

This would be a good time to revisit Chapter Eleven, but restricting your selections to the Breathing category in order to begin slowly. It is definitely going to take time to do it right. So, please S-L-O-W D-O-W-N.

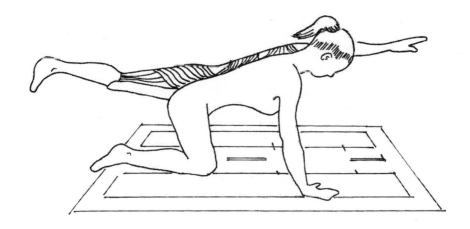

14

THE GOLFER SAYS IT ALL

The Golfer Has Unusual Challenges

Not everyone has the opportunity to celebrate a birthday by playing golf in a recently cut hayfield in Belgrade, Montana. Some of my family members were trying out the game for the first time. None of us was articulating the biomechanics of golf that you might find described in golf magazines or in *Athletic and Sport Issues* in *Musculoseletal Rehabilitation*, where David Lindsay and Anthony A. Vandervoort discuss the biomechanics of golf. But we were enjoying ourselves as we hacked our way through a "golf experience" that was totally in the rough, even the "greens." But so wonderful none the less.

If you play golf, you are experiencing the healthy benefits of playing this popular sport that boasts of approximately 30,000 golf courses and 55 million participants, worldwide. David Lindsay and Anthony Vandervoort have written about the mechanics of the golfswing as well as physical advantages to the golfer who walks a regular eighteen-hole course. For some reason they did not research a course that was carved out of a hayfield in the foothills of Bridger Mountains, Montana. However, if you have an interest in more details covering the finer specifics of playing sports—body

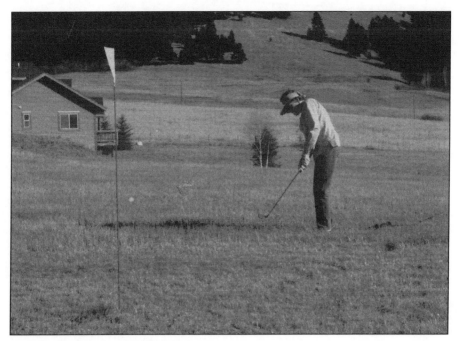
Bridger Mountains Golf Course

movements and muscles that move during your participation — read Chapter Four, "Sports Medicine Board Review." (see Glossary). You will appreciate the exceptional coverage by experts in the medical profession.

Keeping These Considerations in Mind

Getting back to a more ordinary way of life, when listening to your radio do you have a favorite station that plays the kind of music you like to hear? How long has it been since you have heard Norah Jones sing, *Come Away with Me*? Well, I'm asking you to do just that. Come away with me as we go back in time to the 2008 U. S. Open at Torrey Pines, La Jolla, CA. We will relive the lyrics that tell us about pleasant times when people are together. Get set to enjoy the video playback.

I am a volunteer marshal at the eleventh hole on the famous South Course, and we are standing inside the ropes. My assignment is to help manage the crowd. Once everyone stops moving, and silence prevails, we watch each group tee off and come down to the green. This hole is a three-par; therefore, we can watch the pros play their golf ball from tee through the green.

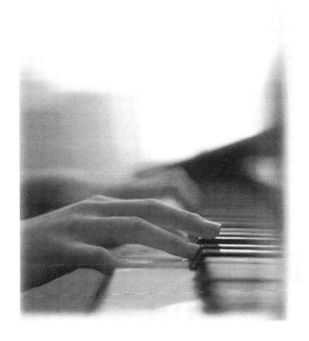

Everyone watching them play was appreciating the blending of kinesthetic and motor dynamics which always occur during such fine specialization of the human musculoskeletal body system. This precision takes place only after thousands of hours are given to cementing such perfection. Certainly, each spectator was appreciating the physiological and mental changes that preceded each golf professional's spectacular control of his mind and body connections.

Watching them, you and I can not help making correlations between the connective dynamics at work, and synchronizing their thoughts with skeletal muscle performance. We are appreciating the many changes that took place in their musculorskeletal system that made such body movements possible.

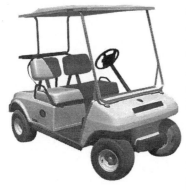

Concepts for Change

In Chapter Four the Concepts for Change give us a structure for making changes in our lives, particularly in our physical and mental form and function. Concepts Two through Six help us associate the changes the professional makes in order to qualify for the U S Open. Since Concept One addresses making improvements, we found no reason to give it our attention.

Concept #2 Positive Direction Comes from Knowledge

Obviously, every pro out there knew a lot about golf and particularly, how to use his skeletal muscles to execute desired finesse and strength. We can see that Rickie Fowler had a plan that included the expert advice from his swing coach, Barry McDonnell. As you recall, I have dedicated this book to Barry because he always, and in all ways, represented how a true golf professional, a teacher and friend, should be.

That day, his prime student was certainly in charge of his game. Rickie's knowledge and thoughts about his game-plan were pretty obvious! It was a treat to see the two of them walking inside the ropes, both realizing their personal **vis vitae**—forces in life, their life ambition.

Rickie Fowler Talks about Barry McDonnell

Later, Rickie took time to make some comments about how Barry talked with him. Barry would encourage him when he was shooting in the low 70's and high 60's, telling him, "You've got 65's in you, Kid." We can appreciate their relationship filled with honor and respect, and why Rickie would later describe Barry saying, "He was always positive and took the highroad… when I would miss hit a shot… he would just tell me to hit another. As he got older he wasn't able to see my ball once it left the clubface, so he would just listen and watch me swing. It always amazed me how much he could tell and help me by just sitting there listening and watching me, and of course on the late afternoons, cigar in hand."

Rick tells us that Barry would say, "Just stay patient, Rick," or "Just go out and play your game."

Concept #3 *Quality Attracts Attention*

We are now getting similar impressions from watching other pros play. This group of professionals was gathered together to demonstrate their exceptional talents, and they certainly were attracting attention. Their presence was closely matching the Concept that covers being organized and being admired for accomplishments. The entire field of players represented this concept, clothed in a stable, yet flexible body structure, they were capable of repeatedly performing flexible muscle movements. I was reminded of Rickie saying that Barry would tell him to, "Just go beat Old Man Par," or to swing easy while keeping his... "left arm just straight and down the line through impact."

Concept #4 *Physical Fitness has an Attitude*

Looking Squared Away is definitely attractive. The players appeared to have that "good feeling" about how they looked and moved. No matter where their ball landed, they walked up to it totally focused on their next shot. I heard no one talk about circumstances causing their ball to land where it did. Those in the foursome had already figured that out.

Concept #5 *Success Breeds Confidence*

The players certainly knew about Self-actualizing Skills, especially self-awareness and self-assessment. Right away we noticed how calm and poised they were. Rick said Barry would tell him to "Just stay patient." Talk about paying attention, they were definitely "in the moment".

Concept #6 *The Squared Away Body is Universally Appealing*

You might have suspected that I would call your attention to their natural posture. Watching the players walk down the fairway or addressing the ball, each one portrayed a classic image—feet pointed straight ahead, head and shoulders in excellent alignment—no extra pounds and mostly looking straight ahead. Talk about a neutral anatomical body posture, they had it!

I hope you enjoyed our short visit to The Open and watching the pros. Now, back to the rest of the book and making some interesting decisions.

The New You

This chapter embraces the New You. Although the content in this chapter has special relevance for the golfer, it is equally important to all readers. Regardless of where you walk — down a fairway, hallway or driveway — or with whom you are meeting, you have an attractive ambiance to carry with you.

The New You slides out of your car more easily and moves with greater confidence, composure and deliberation. You have confidence in the Squared Away principles that have consequence and relevance to maintaining your neutrally anatomical, skeletal muscle performance.

Applying What You Know

Your body relishes the peace and quiet of not having to cope with misalignments or *hidden agenda*. It prefers to move when in a neutral and unstressed condition. You can choreograph desirable muscle movements using kinesthetic awareness as you consciously manage your thoughts — thinking about, remembering what, and analyzing results. Making proper selections from Chapter Fifteen and practicing them on a regular basis, will take you wherever you want to go.

You Are On Your Way

Look often into your mirror. Continue making self-assessments, so you can stay current and recognize changes that need your attention. Set your thoughts on the plan you have for this commitment. Stay committed to the Squared Away seamless design, for reaching and maintaining your *vis vitae*. Focus on appropriate kinesthesia when practicing and during your waking hours.

You can feel good about having traits similar to those of The Thinker—someone who is methodical, a seeker of knowledge and who thinks before taking action.

Congratulations and Play Well!

PRIMED for SQUARE CANONS

Personally Speaking

In the past, I can remember starting my regimen by lying down on my practice mat, watching the news—thinking I was making good use of my time. Actually, my efforts were just the opposite—I remembered little of the news, and included very few Prime Body Canons during my session. Indeed, I was practicing dumb.

Now that times have changed, my *Primed for Square* pages are well worn from rereading the canons once a week as a reminder of how to move and breathe. These are the "prime" areas to "prime".

Prime With Caution

Be reminded that body *strength* appears to be more available in men than women, and *flexibility* is more often available to the female than the male. Also, your progress will be uneven, especially when structural muscles are experiencing specific movements for the first time. Do not be discouraged when occasionally experiencing some "after shocks" and an *atypical* body condition returns. Stay the course and with patience, you can *"fix it."*

Remembering that every exercise is not for everyone, when practicing your body movements, STOP and find another more suited to your physiological needs and condition. Seeking the help and guidance from professionals should always be an alternative now and during the years ahead.

Priming Our Mental Set

During most of our waking hours, whether *prone*, *sitting* or *standing*, we are managing our thoughts in order to move our voluntary muscles as we choose. In addition. many of our involuntary muscles are also helping us carry out our intentions.

As we practice, we are affirming our understanding of the current scientific knowledge of the human body. We can use these advancements to make choices for changing and protecting our body performance and structure.

Three Truths guide our thinking about the tenacious nature of imbalances, and the Concepts for Change guide our choices about muscle performance. With these assets on hand, deciding to make use of them, suggests a lifetime commitment to Whole Body Health practices.

Breathing

Be aware of your breathing techniques when *standing, sitting* or *lying down*.

Although Chapter Eleven reviews the principles for developing breathing skills, maybe you are still wondering— what is the big deal about breathing properly? I refer to Dr. Fellow's explanation about the value of keeping our spine flexible, well nourished and hydrated.

Lubricating your body is such an easy thing to do. It is readily accomplished by simply knowing how to: (1) take air into the lower part of your lungs (2) push your lungs back against your spine and (3) as you hold this alignment, slowly exhaling. Such compression and decompression of the discs allow lengthening in the spinal column as they are hydrated from moisture taken from surrounding tissue. Increasing flexibility is "key" to all musculoskeletal performance.

If you lie down when following these steps, add to the exhaling process, the engagement of your abdominals and tilting your pelvis slightly upward. Classic Pilates breathing suggests breathing through the nose and exhaling from the mouth.

Standing

When the body movement requires you to stand, have your heels even with one another, and toes pointing straight ahead, so there is approximately a space of about four fingers between your two big toes. If this stance is uncomfortable, realign toes until comfortable. Your weight is evenly distributed, yet slightly pitched forward, so you can feel more weight on the balls of your feet, and your heels are pushing into the floor surface.

When the directions do not require movement, tighten your stomach and thigh muscles as you press legs together—as if zipping them tightly so there is no light between them. The entire leg-line is close together up to the pelvic girdle. Bring your hips back and down so they are in line with your ears. In addition, many of our involuntary muscles are also helping us carry out our intentions.

Priming on the Mat the First Few Minutes

After using your line markings and getting set-up on them, begin working with two sets of tennis balls (previously mentioned in Chapter Three) that have been bound together with sturdy tape, such as Duct Tape. Lying down while rolling on the balls, you can locate your "hot spots". When located, place the balls below the "hot spots", and roll back and forth keeping the balls under tissue rather than bone, as you massage the "hot spots", and support your head (hands or a small pillow). You will be amazed at the results.

Practicing Smart

Having decided which body movements to begin experimenting with today, move about your practice area making use of these Primary Constructs for Body Movement.

During every exercise, especially when lying on your mat, keep in mind the natural curvatures of your spine—as you flatten your back on the floor, leaving the spinal curvatures off the surface. Also, check to insure that your body is on the center line and your head is resting on the shoulder and center line intersection.

Enjoy yourself!

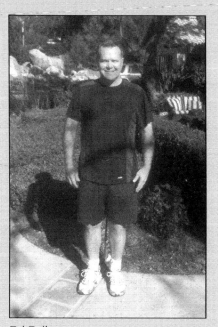

Ed Fellow

15

BODY-MOVEMENTS
TAKE SHAPE

What to Expect

This chapter has illustrations and explanations of body movements to practice. Regardless of how extensive or limited your experience has been with exercising and/or athletic activities, Squared Away technology considers the accomplished athlete, the artisan, as well as the reader, you, who may be for the first time considering musculoskeletal prescriptions. These body movements are a sampling of those I have learned while under the guidance of several professional instructors as well as personal modifications of "old stand bys" which may seem familiar to you.

Each one of us has unique kinesthetic feelings we notice when our muscles move our body parts. Two generic terms are used to describe them: "turned on" and "fired up." You will have your own individual combination of feelings when putting your muscles into this condition. You will also recognize the accomplishment when it happens. Success in making changes in our body alignment depends on being "setup" properly. There are many good CD's and good practioners capable of using these terms well.

Personally Speaking

Over the past few years, trying to solve my postural problems, I have worked with several highly skilled individuals, employees the Egosque Method Headquarters in San Diego, CA, and the Scripps Therapy Clinic, Torrey Pines, La Jolla, CA. (see Bibliography).
I received excellent professional help from both of these health facilities. Included are a few versions of practices that I learned during our time together. Other body movement practices are either those recently learned or developed through my own trial-and-error struggle for physiological improvement.

Then, several years ago I met Kat Folger, a trainer for wellness and rehabilitation. Her physical conditioning theory and her proposal for helping people change their body posture, were the combination for which I had long been searching. I determined that if she could truly apply her words of wisdom to improve my body condition, I would absorb all she would provide. Kat has been exceptionally helpful because she individualized her expertise to meet my unique physiological needs. I am no longer minimizing the damage caused by kyphosis and scoliosis — I am now focusing on improvement.

Kat's latest summary of my postural disruptions indicated that no one would ever know that I had damage from kyphosis. There was also a bonus in being her student. Meeting Monday mornings at the Hilltop Center, in Fallbrook, CA, with like-minded men and women on their practice mats, representing all age groups (teen to eighty) is my real inspiration. This, in itself, is healing; but sharing usually is.

Listening In

Before moving on, read these comments as I address a few good friends and treasured family members who have resisted conducting a thorough Self-awareness and Self-assessment Examination.

It☐s Never Too Late!

Dear Family and Friends,

I just wanted to tell you that I had your back when writing and choosing the information to include in Squared Away. Truly, this book can help you fit wonderful Whole Life practices into 4 or 5 hours a week. And get this, you can do it without leaving your home in order to take advantage of an improved life style. You can set your own schedule. You can improve and stabilize your body posture and performance. You can select body movements designed for your special body structure. How can you resist such sensible reassurances which can turn heads toward you now as well as in the years to come?

Because you often ask me about my golf game, and laugh with me about some of the weird shots I make out on the course, all I can say right now is that the ball is no longer veering left, and I have much more confidence in my swing. When I finish writing this book, I will get serious about lowering my handicap—of course, using the Concepts for Change.

Best wishes, Mary.

I know you are anxious to select your body movements. Now that you know which body parts you want to improve, consider which ones you want to practice. Have fun!

SELECTING BODY MOVEMENT PRACTICES

Make use of your recorded body measurements. Since the words, "no pain, no gain," are no longer valued, "taking it easy" are very acceptable replacements. So, take a leisurely tour through this sampling of body movements while thinking about which ones will be the right ones for meeting your skeletal muscle needs. Here is an example of matching misalignments with body movement practices.

Example

Suppose you have a right hip misaligned. It is positioned forward of the left hip, and throwing your whole body posture off-center. Your corrective measures would include practicing Breathing Principles as you work with other body movement exercises to help correct postural problems. You may need to bring a hip or shoulder back into the socket— pushing it down, back and inward toward your **center line**, or **median line**. Focus should be given to developing a kinesthetic feeling for this rotation so you can repeat it more easily. Check to see that you have not caused misalignments in other parts of your body when practicing these body movements.

ROLLING ON TENNIS BALLS (1)

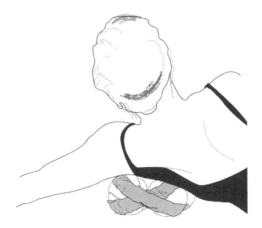

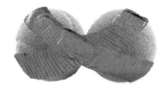

Starting Position

Lying down on your back.

Purpose

Relaxing your back, shoulder and leg muscles.

Action

Using your four tennis balls (two sets that have been bound together with sturdy tape, such as Duct Tape, or put into a sock for more comfort), roll on the balls, supporting your head with your hands or using a small pillow. Move your body over them to discover your "hot spots." You are cautioned about keeping the balls on tissue *not* bone and supporting your head while rolling on your back. Don't hurt yourself. Now, place the balls below the "hot spots" and roll back and forth, keeping the balls under tissue rather than bone, as you massage the sensitive areas. Relax a few moments before beginning other body movement exercises.

More Advanced

This is all you need to do with the tennis balls until you find another means for loosening up your body parts.

ROTATING ANKLE AND FOOT CIRCLES (2)

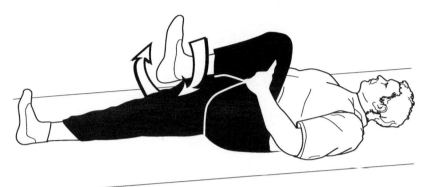

Starting Position

Lying down on your back, establish Squared Away position on your mat; especially, matching your heels with the **mat heel markings**. Head is in proper position so you can stretch neck muscles and create a thinner chest.

Purpose

This exercise is less intense than others. It strengthens tissue and muscles important to supporting our body and its movement when using them (walking, standing, etc).

Action

1. While lying on your back, be sure your core muscles are "turned on" before extending both legs and your toes pointed toward the ceiling

2. Roll your hips backward and down into the mat surface; after positioning these muscles and body parts, somewhat tilt your pelvis

3. Bend one leg toward your chest and support it by clasping your hands behind the knee and keeping muscles in your thighs pulled down and heavy

onto the mat surface with shoulders deep into their sockets

4. Begin by first bending your ankle so that your toes are pointing toward the ceiling. Then relaxing—bend your ankle so that the angle between the sole of your foot is increased then decreased (dorsiflexion)

5. Now, you can more easily circle your foot by rotating your ankle and keeping the knee still so that the foot is being moved only by the ankle (not by the knee) Begin circling the foot, and flexing it toward your body

6. You will feel tension in your leg and foot muscles, the toes are not collapsed

7. Change legs and repeat several times on each side—breathing slowly, easily and fully

More Advanced

Continue bringing the bent leg closer to your chest. Do not over extend, stay comfortable.

STRETCHING AND BENDING UPPER TORSO (3)

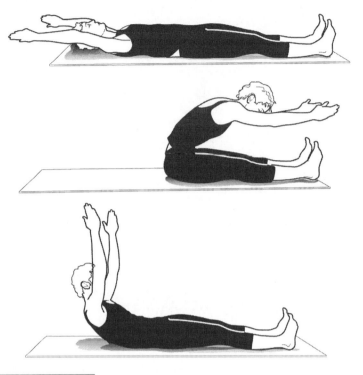

Starting Position

You are lying down with your back on your mat. These body movements are not for the Beginner, they can be beneficial to the Intermediate and Advanced student. You need to have control of your back and neck muscles when raising and lowering your body off the mat.

Purpose

When breathing correctly, this group of body movements can be very helpful. Because muscles in and around decompressed vertebrae are more easily manipulated, greater gains can be realized in lengthening your spinal column, thus relieving aches and pains. Before attempting the exercises, think about gently lengthening the neck, and the space above the ears, without moving your shoulders out of position, and by keeping them down into their sockets during these body movements.

1. Lying down, facing the ceiling, legs are straight out, and toes are flexed, pointing straight up toward the ceiling, arms are stretched out behind your head alongside your ears with palms facing in and when air enters lower lobes of the lungs, your ribs will expand and push down into the floor surface

2. Stabilize your shoulders—rounding them down into their sockets pushing them gently into the mat along with your scapulae

3. Exhaling, keep your abdominals engaged, begin rolling your torso upward as one unit so that your arms come to position beside your ears as you rise up off the mat surface

4. Your torso and arms stretch toward your feet and at the same time, your neck and head are raised into position so you can look through this opening and can see your feet

5. As you continue bending forward, articulating your vertebrae one-at-a-time off the mat surface, your head stays between the arms without dropping your chin to your chest

6. When your arms are stretched out over your legs, your torso is bent over your legs and your arms are parallel to the floor

7. Briefly holding this position, inhale and rest a few seconds, as you exhale, articulate vertebrae one-at-a-time back onto mat surface while keeping arms alongside your ears and shoulders relaxed as much as possible

8. Maintain natural spinal curvatures as you relax and return to original position, repeating 5–10 times

More Advanced

Work at progressively lengthening your arms and torso over your legs—increasing distance between vertebra without disturbing the body movements recommended.

STRENGTHEN GLUTES (4)

Pelvic Girdle: includes sacrum, hip
and femur

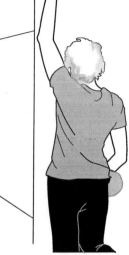

Starting Position

You will be standing with right side
about the width of your fist away from
a wall. This is one of my favorites
because it seems so simple, yet you
can get a lot accomplished.

Purpose

This exercise helps strengthen muscles
in the hip area. Improvement in your balance
can also occur.

Action

1. Hold the body in the Squared Away position and
   right side about a fist-width away from the wall,
   bring your left foot as close to the right foot as
   possible without changing your posture

2. Place a folded towel or 7- or 8-inch ball between
   the upper part of hip bone and the wall, keeping
   body in aligned position; you may feel a burning
   sensation in the standing hip

3. Keeping shoulders and all other body parts from
   moving, bend inside leg at knee so that toes are
   pointing down toward floor surface while ever-so-
   slightly, rolling the right hip so that the ball rises
   no more than1/2 to 2 inches

4. Continue this small hip movement keeping ears
   above shoulders with eyes looking straight ahead

5. Repeat 5–10 times, then change sides

More Advanced

Raise arm on outside of body toward the ceiling, keeping the
arm alongside your ear and palm facing inward.

SHOULDER, ARM and NECK (5)

Shoulder Rolls

Starting Position

Standing in front of a wall and, if possible, in front of a mirror. Of course, establish your neutral anatomical or Squared Away body posture.

Purpose

While your muscles are in neutral position, roll your shoulder to strengthen and stretch these muscles, thus making them more flexible.

Action

Shoulder rolls may not seem important, but when shoulder muscles are rotated appropriately, our whole body benefits.

1. Stand against a wall with your head, upper back and hips against the wall, spinal curvatures respected, feet are shoulder-width apart and away from wall by a few inches, buttocks and calves are touching the wall and heels close to it

2. Bring your shoulder blades (scapulae) closer together without moving your head

3. Slowly roll your shoulders backward and down— maintaining the Squared Away posture throughout the rest of your body

4. Relax your shoulders and reposition for repeating these muscle movements

5. Reverse direction if appropriate, repeating throughout the day when possible

More Advanced

Practice these body movements when not against a wall and are maintaining a neutral anatomical body posture and balance. Accomplishing these shoulder movements occurs by just staying with the fundaments; they are sufficient.

CHILD'S POSE (6)

Stretches ankles, hips and upper torso muscles

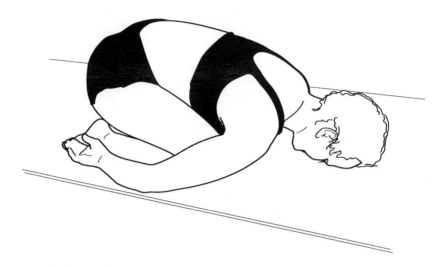

Starting Position

Begin by kneeling down and facing the floor. This is a good stretching and resting position. However, this exercise is not as easily accomplished by men because they tend to be less flexible in the spine, hips and shoulders than women. Do not use this exercise if you find it uncomfortable. however, if you want to try, the steps to take are below.

Purpose

With practice, shoulders become less rigid, back muscles and upper legs more flexible.

Action

You are probably familiar with this pose. It is very popular and quite worth the credits given.

1. To get set-up, your knees are bent on the practice mat, and buttocks are resting on your heels and if possible—while aligning knees, ankles and toes—form a straight line as you leave space between the thighs so your chest can rest between your legs

2. Bend body so that your chin is tucked inward, your arms are stretched back and out alongside your body with palms facing up toward the ceiling

3. Hold for several minutes, relaxing your shoulders down while all other body parts are at rest

More Advanced

This is not an exercise that deserves more intensity. Keeping the body relaxed and flexible during the movements is the goal.

HAMSTRING, INNER THIGH and SHOULDER STRENGTHENING (7)

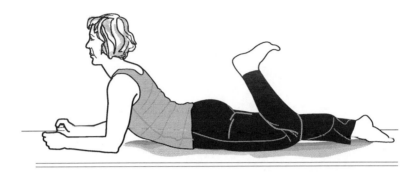

Starting Position

Lying face down, here is a version of Single-Leg Kick. I have practiced these body movements for many years, but correctly learned them from reading C. Murakami's book (see Bibliography).

Purpose

Strengthening hamstrings. Take your time learning to use these body movements because muscles and the vertebra in our lower spines need to learn slowly. Stop if stress or pain occurs. Body parts are heavy on the mat surface.

Action

1. Lying on your stomach, your upper torso is supported by your elbows and your hands are made into fists, raise your "abs" up off the floor

and hamstrings are contracting—core muscles are "turned on"

2. Your legs are extended in straight line, and feet about 3–5 inches apart; while keeping your head and neck in line with your spine, inhale and bend one knee, flexing it toward the buttocks, 2–3 times

3. Exhale and lower the leg to starting position, then inhale and raise other leg alternating for several minutes

4. Focus on breathing correctly as you time your leg movements accordingly

More Advanced

Do not add more to these body movements.

STRETCHING CALF and HAMSTRINGS (8)

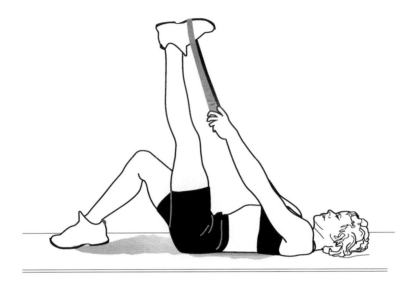

Lie down on your back using a band or towel to stretch legs.

Purpose

This exercise works with your arms and legs while engaging the "powerhouse" which is composed of the abdominal muscles, hips, lower back muscles and buttocks.

Action

Using the markings on your mat will keep you squared.

1. Right leg is bent for support, with sole of foot on mat surface and arms are stretched out alongside, but not touching your body

2. A band or towel is wrapped around the sole of your foot, and leg is pulled straight up keeping the leg firmly stretched and directly over the body with the sole of the foot parallel to the floor— optimum range of leg is when the foot reaches placement over your head

3. While pulling band taut and, without loosing natural spinal curvatures, keep your hips and spine on the mat surface (respecting natural spinal curvatures) and pulling toes down toward your left hip to feel stretch in back of left leg

4. The entire "powerhouse" is "turned on" (includes abdominal muscles, lower back muscles, our hips and buttocks)

5. Stay in the Squared Away position and hold 10–20 seconds so you can feel the "pull" in your leg muscles, then gently bring the leg back to original position

6. Rest and change legs; repeat directions for opposite leg

More Advanced

When comfortable, increase the angle at which your leg is pulled by extending it in a higher arc toward your head, while keeping abdominals firm and spine flat on the floor.

PELVIC and SHOULDER-BRIDGING (9)

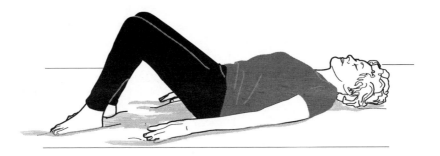

Starting Position

Lying on your back, knees are bent and feet are flat on mat surface.

Purpose

These body movements might seem to be easily accomplished. If practiced correctly, they can become one of the "basic movements" to use daily for developing control of your body performance and function. You can work on improving the flexibility and strength of your shoulder and arm muscles by using them during these muscle movements.

Action

Align your body using the center, shoulder and heel lines on your mat. Arms are placed alongside your body with palms down.

1. As you exhale, tighten glutes and tilt your hips slightly upward while keeping your arms, head, upper part of your shoulders and feet on the mat

2. While your buttocks and hips are elevated and muscles in pelvic area are tightened (squeezing buttocks) roll your shoulders slightly under you as pictured in the illustration

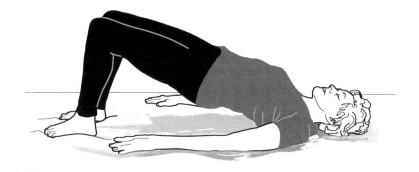

3. Keeping cervical vertebrae on surface, elevate your breastbone toward your chin and feel the pressure coming from pushing the balls of your feet and your arms down into mat surface

4. After taking several breaths, exhale and begin to slowly bring your body back to starting position as you articulate your vertebrae one-by-one back onto the floor surface

5. Repeat and continue to synchronize breathing with action

More Advanced

Increase number of repetitions and try tapping the palms of your hands up and down on the floor surface. While breathing during pumping motion use 5 counts inhaling and exhaling while tightening muscles in your core. Repeat as often as is comfortable.

SQUATS (10)

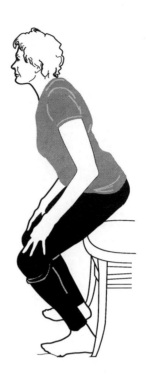

Starting Position

Sit in a chair or on a bench with a band tightly stretched just below the knees.

Purpose

Developing flexibility and strength of the glutes and leg muscles helps with controlling your musculoskeletal body parts in the Squared Away body structure. This exercise helps align hips as you"turn on" your glutes and tighten muscles in the front of your upper leg.

Action

Have available a towel or band and a chair.

1. Stretch the towel or/ band around both legs just below knees, legs are straight against the band, tighten it so it is taut, then place your hands on your knees—keeping your back straight and head in line with shoulders—especially keeping your chin in while looking straight ahead

2. Sitting on edge of chair with hips rolled backward, push your tailbone out and back—giving an arch to your lower back—as you place your feet hip-width apart with toes straight ahead

3. Tighten correction areas and rise up off the chair seat 8–10 inches while maintaining the original position—semi-sitting position

4. Without sitting down, return body to level just above seat; continue bobbing up and down while keeping your neutral alignment, repeating as many times as comfortable. If you have *atypical* knees or back, do not use this body movement

More Advanced

Increase band tightness, also adding more pressure when pushing legs against the band. Gradually add horizontal squats with your back on the floor and feet against the wall.

SIDE BRACING PLANK (11)

Most of the musculoskeletal system

Lying on stomach, with feet flexed and up against a wall. I began practicing this body movement, using a wall to support my body, until I could go it alone. Here are the steps to take when beginning.

Purpose

You will be working on body alignment, stretching and balancing as you stack your body on each side.

Action

Take time to get your body aligned and set. Conduct this exercise with your legs stretched out, with feet against a wall or door and lying on your stomach.

1. Lie down with arms in prayer position, your elbows are under shoulders, legs stretched out and feet together with soles of feet pushing against the wall

2. When balanced, twist your body and stack your left foot on top of the right, feet are together up against the wall; now, flex both with the outside edge of the right foot firmly pushing into the wall and floor—supporting the shift in body weight

3. As you rotate your body, your right arm is bent and has turned laterally, pointing away from your body—still at shoulder height—supporting the side-bracing alignment where all body parts are elevated in a straight line off the floor except for the edge of the right foot and ankle and your right arm (still bent at 90 degrees)

4. Abdominals, lower glutes, inner thighs and hamstrings are all "engaged" so that your body is in a straight line from head to the soles of your

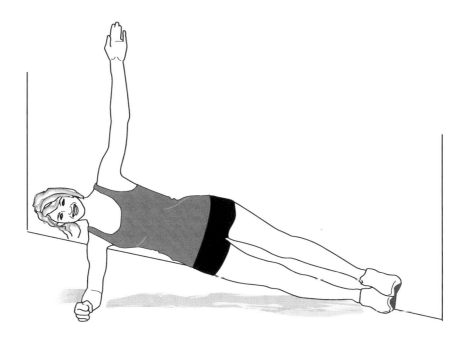

feet and forming Squared Away body alignment
(transversely) and (coronally) from forehead to
center of flexed sole of your feet

5. Hold for 10–20 seconds, adjusting torso so that it
    is aligned (not caved in) with the rest of your body

6. Exhaling, return to original position with arms in
    prayer position under shoulders

7. Rest and breathe for a minute or two then change
    sides

More Advanced

After your muscles are strong enough to eliminate using a
wall to brace your rotation, make these body movements as
outlined. Also, try raising your outside arm above your head.
It should be in a straight line with your body, especially in the
mid-section where alignment "cave-in" can happen. Hold
position for 30–60 seconds, change sides, using 2:1 ratio for
side needing more care.

WALL PRESS (12)

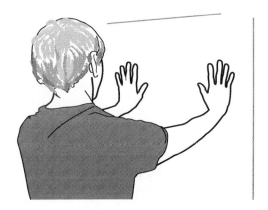

Starting Position

Standing

Purpose

Strengthing shoulder girdle and core while working on your shoulder, elbows, wrists and fingers to strengthen a Squared Away body posture.

Action

The action in the body is centered in the shoulders, your back and through the arms and wrists.

1. Stand facing a wall with your body assuming the Pilates Stance and your hips rolled down and inward—directly below shoulders that are back and rolled down into their sockets—legs are relaxed and knees are not locked

2. Place your hands on the wall by separating each finger and thumb, spreading them out on the wall with elbows extended, palms of hands are flat against the wall

3. Without shoulders moving, use your arms to exert pressure and push against the wall, keeping muscles in upper core "turned on" and alignment unaltered when forcing pressure on the wall

4. Hold for 30 seconds. repeat 10–15 times

More Advanced

Change the position of your palms by pointing fingers more toward the side or facing downward. Also begin translating these movements into those involved when doing push-ups.

CLIMBER (13)

Strengthens Muscles Bilaterally

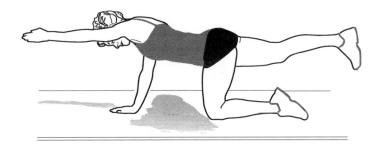

Starting Position

Kneel down while alternating stretching of each extended arm.

Purpose

This exercise specializes in helping our musculoskeletal system work with flexibility, strength and balance. The whole chain of muscles and bones on each side of your body is engaged during this body movement.

Action

This exercise is well known, and when correctly practiced, can quite effectively accomplish a variety of physiological needs by alternating arm and leg pose. The key to gaining help from it, is in staying in alignment on your mat.

1. With your body centered on **center line**, kneel so that your hands are below your shoulders, your knees are directly below your hips, and wrists are bent with fingers extending from the palm of your hand

2. Muscles are tightened and back is leveled with the Squared Away alignment in place

3. When balanced, lift and straighten one leg while stretching an arm on the alternate side of your body—straight out in front of you with palm facing inward and parallel to mat surface

4. Now, you have a single leg (knee bent) and opposite arm supporting your body (see illustration)

5. Keep your back and shoulder muscles "fired up" as you hold this pose, repeat 2 times, alternating between sides

More Advanced

Depending on side needing more strength and/or balance, use the 1:2 ratio (double time on the area needing more help) increasing strength of the muscles "turned on".

GROUNDED TORSO POSE (14)

Stretching and training core and leg muscles

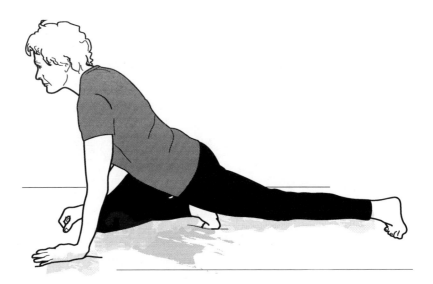

Starting Position

Kneeling down with one leg stretched out, the other bent and the elbow pushing into it. Positioning for making these body movements is rather difficult at first, but worth the time spent when accomplished.

Purpose

I designed this exercise to bilaterally stretch my hip, and shoulder muscles while improving ability to adequately "turn on" my inner core.

Action

Assume the body positions as illustrated, you will be working on hip alignment and leg stretches.

1. Start in a kneeling (quadruped) position, while on your hands and knees, stretch left leg straight out behind your left hip and at the same time supporting yourself with the bent right knee and hand

2. Now, slide the left leg farther behind you while bending the right knee as much as possible so that the right forearm can rest on this thigh (see illustration)

3. Pointing left foot and leg straight behind you so that the toes of the foot are on the mat surface with the palm of your left hand directly under your left shoulder

4. Leaning slightly forward, keeping balance with left hand on floor surface, inhale and push the bottom side of your bent right forearm into your right thigh

5. As you maintain this pose, breathing with short breaths, use a deep massaging motion with your forearm, continue applying pressure to this thigh

6. Keep the muscles in your "powerhouse" (abdominal muscles, hips, lower back muscles and buttocks) "fired up," take several breaths and come back to normal

7. Switch legs

More Advanced

I often perform these body movements during my exercise program, especially after practicing body movements that stretch the leg muscles and need a rest. Advanced action would be to raise and lower your hip bones without moving your body while in the squatting position.

MIRROR REACHES (15)

Standing in front of mirror

Muscles in upper torso

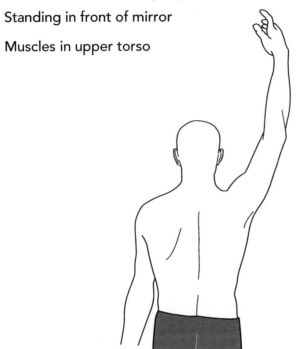

Stand facing a mirror.

Purpose

This is an exercise for correcting/improving misalignments caused by scoliosis and/or kyphosis.

Action

The purpose is to bring the asymmetrical spinal alignment, which is inherent with scoliosis, into better alignment BEFORE strengthening muscles associated with this problem. You will be raising one arm at-a-time above your head aligning with your ears, training muscles in your shoulders to fall back and into their sockets. This does not seem too difficult, nor is it. However, if all the alignment strategies can take place when raising and keeping the arm as well as the rest of the body aligned correctly, this is an accomplishment.

1. Stand facing a mirror using heel lines on mat and checking your balance, adjust stance if necessary, begin using muscles in your arms to roll muscles in the shoulder core back toward spine and down into your shoulder sockets, while also "turning on" muscles required when taking the Pilates Stance which includes:

2. Engaging the core and shoulder blades, so that the shoulder girdle is stable and firm

3. Now, raise left arm pushing it down towards your collarbone, without bending your elbow, and keeping it alongside your ear while looking straight ahead

4. Head is being pushed back so the ears are above the shoulders

More Advanced

Advancements come when your body alignment takes shape in the ideal Squared Away or Pilates Stance, and aligning without strain.

HUNDRED (16)

Arms, core and legs

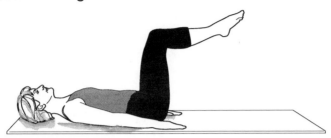

Starting Position

Although the Hundred is taught, practiced and included in many physiological regimen these body movements are not easily mastered. This exercise is too difficult for the Beginner in its original form. These body movements have been modified to accommodate less demands on our physicality.

Purpose

The Hundred is practiced to firm the body's core as well as tone the upper leg muscles.

Action

Begin lying with your back on the mat, with your legs in the air and your calves are parallel to the mat surface—forming an "L"—and the arms are resting alongside your body with palms down. Your abs are "on fire" the entire time and all surrounding tissue "turned on."

1. Legs remain in tabletop with toes pointing toward the ceiling, but ankles are somewhat relaxed as your pelvis is in neutral position—tucked—stretch your arms toward your feet, keeping the space between your hips and ribs firm so they do not collapse

2. As you lie on your mat, take a few breaths, then when exhaling, stretch your legs straight out (to about a 45 degree angle) while raising your upper

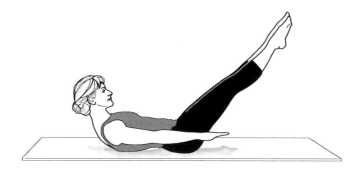

torso forward; this is a smooth movement made without jerking or pulling your head forward or to one side

3. Your arms are raised several inches off the floor while simultaneously lifting your head and shoulders off the mat, do not tuck your chin into your chest or permit your feet to flop backward

4. Maintain this posture as you pump your arms up and down in rhythm—inhaling for 5 counts and exhaling for 5 counts

5. Exhaling, slowly return to beginning position, repeat several times, keeping the pelvis area neutrally positioned with scapula down and back when returning to the mat surface

6. By keeping your eyes on your inner thighs as you raise and lower your head, better alignment can be maintained

More Advanced

As mentioned above, this set of body movements is one of the more difficult to perform. I have been working on this particular set for a year, and still have not mastered the complexity of it. It is included because some of you are Intermediate or Advanced and might want another description of it. In addition. Pilates instructors can offer expert advice on the muscle movements required.

FINDING BALANCE (17)

Stand close to a wall or any surface you can touch with your hand for support. Take the steps slowly. Finding one's balance with eyes open is a challenge; finding it with eyes closed, will take some time.

Purpose

Closing our eyes and finding our balance gets us in touch with our inner core.

Action

1. Take the Pilates Stance (page 97), close your eyes and find your balance; keeping eyes closed put your hand on the wall for stability

2. Focusing on the muscles and alignments necessary for maintaining a well aligned body structure, try maintaining this posture for a few seconds at a time until no support is needed

3. When comfortable with this posture, slowly bend one knee and lift one foot off the floor surface (about 2–4 inches)

3. Keep contact with your support and try to maintain the lifted foot with eyes closed and gradually you will be able to perform these balancing techniques without support

More Advanced

The goal is to reach the point where you can perform these body movements with eyes closed and without needing to support yourself while maintaining your balance for 30–60 seconds, and with one foot raised for 10–30 seconds.

You may also use a phone book, block, or lifts to stand on and add alternate movements by changing positions of one leg and then the other.

TOTAL RELAXATION FOR EVERYONE (18)

Fifteen Minutes of Peace and Quiet

Starting Position

Lying down: whenever you can take 15 minutes to improve your sense-of-humor, make use of this approach. I learned it while taking lessons from Egosque (see Bibliography).

Purpose

Relaxing our entire body in this position allows the muscles to release tension, especially in the vertebra area.

Action

Getting set and letting your muscles relax is the only action required. Practicing this form of involuntary body movements should be one of everyone's choices.

1. Tuck your mat along the foot line under a cushion on a standard-height chair and stretch the rest of your mat out in front of the chair

2. Lying down, place the back of your head on the safety pins or Scotch-tape—the intersection of the center line and head line—stretch your legs out, with heels on the chair cushion

3. The center of your body should be on the center line as you relax your arms and remain unmoving in this position for about 10–15 minutes

4. Roll to the side and gently come to sitting then standing, feel how relaxed your muscles are while at the same time more flexible

5. No one needs to tell you about repetitions. Hopefully, you will manage them several times a week

ENJOY!

16

YOU, THE INDIVIDUAL, TAKE RESPONSIBILITY

Achieving such independence comes from having a broadly-based and easily interpreted foundation of reliable information. Squared Away was designed, not only to serve as reminders, but also to increase your understanding of being the self-manager of your physical fitness. In all probability, as you applied knowledge and participated in activities during your read, you were comfortable because the Concepts for Change were there, keeping you going "full circle" on the Squared Away ride of Achievement.

Recognizing Progress

One can not help but notice the outstanding accomplishments you have made while you were improving and maintaining your Whole Body Health condition through repetition. This posture should be your inspiration for completing a body condition that manifests flexibility, energy and aesthetic movement. Climb aboard and find a seat on the Squared Away Ferris wheel as it constantly carries you around the circle of Repetitive Accomplishments.

Accomplishments to Build On

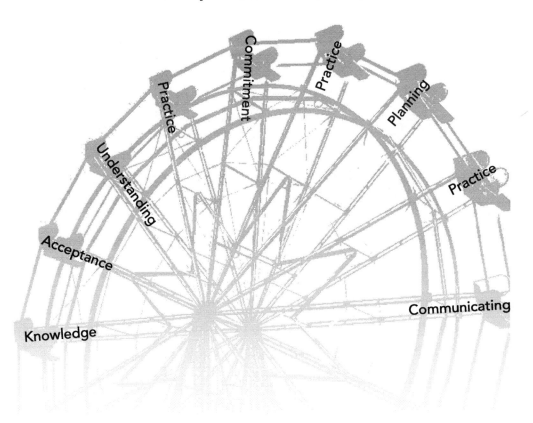

Circle the platform often.

Accomplishments to Build On

You have accepted the Three Truths and the "mind-over-matter syndrome," while using the Three Questions as directives when choosing your **vis vitae**, as you participated in Self-awareness and Self-assessment Skills and projects.

You have knowledge of skeletal muscles, their composition and function; and can translate knowledge of biology and physiology into Practical Applications.

Understanding scientific accomplishments and the contributions stemming from them, have enriched your Self-actualizing Skills, making use of Concepts for Change and interpretations of kinesthesia.

Practicing self-awareness and thought management along with body movement practices such as breathing, taking a stance, etc., has prepared you well for self-actualizing a plan for maintenance.

Having at your disposal vocabulary describing directional planes in which the body moves along with the directions of muscle movement, makes communicating with others quite natural.

Descriptions and illustrations of muscle movement practice, along with an understanding of procedures for working out, bring you into realistic contact with reclaiming and rejuvenating your body's efficiency, effectiveness and attractive characteristics.

You should become a "creature of habit" — making use of the Squared Away Ferris wheel ride — while circling the platform often.

Let's Get Squared Away

Proper Body Alignments, A Working Definition—The human body is aligned when the shoulders, hips and knees are aligned within 1/2 inch of identified Body Points.

Please respond **to the following based on your opinions, knowledge and/or experience.**

No.	Statements	Yes	No	Comments (use back side if needed)
1.	Body misalignments can describe bodies having mild to severe structural deviations, misshaped bones, body development irregularities, or being temporarily out-of-alignment.			
2.	Many people such as professional athletes, fashion models, people regulary on TV or in the public eye are good practitioners for keeping their bodies Well-Aligned while others may ignore how their bodies "line-up." Have you ever personally been interested in knowing about your Body Alignment as far as having shoulders, hips, and knees showing equal distance from one **body point** such as, earlobes?			
3.	Since everyone has some imperfection in Body Alignment, it is certain that everyday during our daily activities, such as: walking, resting, coping with tired muscles, etc. (exercising excluded) we are constantly repeating certain muscle patterns. These repetitive muscle movements can actually groove misalignment without our being aware we are doing so.			
4.	Some people, believing their **exercise schedule** to be beneficial, may be practicing certain Body Movements incorrectly because they either haven't properly identified their misalignments or didn't know how to treat them. Under these conditions, practice, can actually reinforce misalignment. Knowing how to make a Self-assessment can be helpful in avoiding this error.			
5.	One procedure for conducting a Body Alignment Self-assessment is to take measurements and compare them bilaterally (side-to-side) etc. These measurements can be useful in interpreting differences in Body Alignment from side-to-side and front-to-back.			
6.	One identification of misalignments is recognized using the neutral anatomical body structure. The prescription for selected Body Movements can be made with improved confidence using **body points** that pin-point individual body deviations.			
7.	Awareness of the unique Body Movements in which an individual can engage, should **precede** making selections of Body Movements designed to meet body reshaping or strengthening.			
8.	Advantage in having a balanced Postural Alignment** can be related to having a positive self-image. Similarly, codependence exists between having a Well-Aligned body and those Body Movements athletes practice when perfecting their skills.			

*Neutral anatomical body structure also defines having a Squared Away body alignment.
**Postural Alignment includes having body points within 1/2" of being Squared side-to-side and front-to-back.

GLOSSARY

Acromion comes from the Greek "akron", peak + "omos", shoulder the peak of the shoulder. The acromion acts as an attachment for the muscles that move the shoulder. It articulates with the clavicle to form the acromioclavicular joint, forming the highest point of the shoulder.

Anatomy- the science of dealing with structure of animals and plants.

Antagonist Muscles are a group of muscles that act in opposition to a specific movement made by an agonist.

> **Agonist** is a muscle that causes action.

> **Synergist** describes a muscle that assists another muscle to accomplish movement.

Aponeurosis is a broad flat sheet of dense caliginous connective tissue that serves as a tendon to bind muscles together or to attach muscles to other tissue or bone.

Articular (hyaline) Crtilage- structureless, transparent substance that covers the articular surfaces of bone.

Biochemistsry describes the science of dealing with the chemistry of living matter.

Biology- the study of life or living matter in all of its forms.

Body points- are the spots made during your self-assessment on your shoulders, hips and forehead. They help you to tattoo your mat and define your body balances and imbalances.They are described in Chapter Two.

Core- is used to describe the lumbopelvic and hip complex. The center of gravity is located here and this is the location from where all movement is navigated. The four core muscles: diaphragm, transversus abdominis, multifidus and pelvic floor comprise the inner unit that surrounds the lumbar spine and pelvis.

Descriptions of Human Muscle Movements describe different muscle movements when moving appendages and other body-parts such as rolling our hips and shoulders, pointing our feet outward or inward or the movement of our hands and fingers. Below are specific names of muscle movements.

Abduction and **Adduction**- indicate muscle movements taking an appendage away (laterally) from the body center line or toward the frontal plane, respectively.

Extension and **flexion**- Extension is the action of moving a limb from a bent to a straight position or moving body part further apart, whereas flexion moves body parts closer together or is the action of bending or the condition of being bent, especially the bending of a limb or joint.

Circumduction- defines a circular movement that combines flexion, extension, adduction, and abduction without shaft rotation.

Eversion- takes place when moving the sole of foot away from medial plane.

Hyperextension- extends the joint beyond the neutral anatomical position.

Inversion- moves the sole of foot toward the medial plane.

Pronation- involves an internal rotation resulting in appendage facing downward.

Protrusion- involves moving anteriorly (e.g., pushing chest out).

Supination: External rotation resulting in appendage facing upward.

Retrusion: Moving posteriorly (e.g., chin in).

Directional terms are referenced using the following:

Anterior (ventral) and **Posterior (dorsal)**- refer to near to or at the front of the body, and structures nearer to or at the back of the body, respectively.

Superior (crainial) and **Inferior (caudal)**- refer to toward the head or the upper part of the body, and nearer to or at the back of the body, respectively.

Ipsilateral and **Contralateral**- mean on the same side, and on the opposite side of the body structure, respectively.

Medial and **Lateral**- refer to being closer to, and away from the mid line of the body, respectively.

Proximal and **Distal**- identify body structures that are nearer to, and farther from the attachment of an extremity, respectively.

Superficial and **Deep**- direct us toward the surfaces of the body, and away from the surfaces, respectively.

Exercise- this word originated from the Latin root meaning to maintain, keep guard of; we use the word to describe, improve or put into action.

Fascia- is a band or sheath of connective tissue investing, supporting, or binding internal organs, muscles, bones, blood vessels and nerves of the body; sometimes described as a layer of fibrous tissue that acts as a shock absorber in the body.

Hidden agenda- in this text refers to the unnatural reactions our tissue experience when pressure is applied.

Hot spots- are the areas in our muscles where pain is noticed when pressure is applied.

Ilium- comes from Latin meaning groin. The ilium is the uppermost and largest bone in the pelvis.

Kinesiology is the science dealing with the interrelationship of the physiological processes and anatomy of the human body with respect to movement.

Kinesthesia is the sensation of movement or strain in human muscles, tendons and joints—also referred to as muscle sense— that can detect body position, weight and/or movement of the skeletal muscles.

Ligaments connect bones with bones, and are described as fibrous bands or sheets of connective tissue that link two or more structures together.

Musculoskeletal System- provides form, stability and movement for the human body. It is made up of the body's bones, muscles and surrounding tissue.

Myofascia- comes from two Latin words "myo" for muscle and "fascia" for bands. It is often defined as a fibrous tissue that encloses and separates layers of muscles. It is viewed as a body-wide connection among muscles within the fascia net.

Myology- is the branch of biology studying muscles.

Neurolgy- the branch of medicine dealing with the nervous system.

Neuron- is an electrically excitable cell that processes and transmits information by electrical and chemical signaling.

Neutral Anatomical Body Structure- describes a body posture having the same qualifications as the Squared Away body condition. The alignment and function of the skeletal body muscles perform without strain or atypical body conditions.

Neutral anatomical body structure or **neutral posture** is defined as the well aligned body structure when the joints are not bent and the spine is aligned. Also known as being **Squared Away**.

Nervous System- is a complex system of nerves and nerve centers, including the brain, spinal cord, nerves and ganglia. Used when referring to animals and humans, often used to explain interactions between the body and its adjustments to the environment.

Periosteum- is the membrane covering the external surface of bone, enabling tendons to establish connection with the surface of bone.

Physical Fitness- for this manuscript, represents the Squared Away body condition—not exceeding ½ inch variation between each body point when compared with the partner.

Physiology- is a branch of biology dealing with the functions and activities of living organisms and their parts.

Physiotherapy- studies body movements in terms of neurophysiology and mechanical aspects, which help in the interpretation of the actual mechanisms of movement.

Powerhouse of the Body Structure- in the Pilates method, refers to the combination of abdominal muscles, hips, the lower back muscles and buttocks.

Types of Human Muscles:

> **Smooth Muscle-** describes the muscles that surround organs and tissue. They are involuntary muscles and found in blood vessels, organs and other life-sustaining tissue.

> **Heart Muscle-** is found only in the heart.

> **Skeletal Muscle-** is a voluntary muscle that moves and supports the skeleton, found in muscles associated with the body movement.

Vis vitae- vis in Latin means: strength, force and power. *Vitae* is Latin meaning curriculum. *Vis vitae*, therefore, defines the energy of life, and a constant force that gives energy and keeps us going.

Whole Body Health- considers all aspects of improving, maintaining and specializing the human body efficiency and effectiveness. It takes place when we are: Taking a Proper Stance, Breathing Correctly and Self-managing Our Thoughts.

BIBLIOGRAPHY

Whenever needed, throughout the text *Random House Webster's Unabridged Dictionary, Second Edition*, and *Wikipedia* were used to clarify and explain language and references, **not** context, in the book.

Begley, Sharon with Ian Yarett. "Can You Build a Stronger Brain?" *Newsweek Magazine.* January 10 &17, 2011.

Brynie, Faith Hickman, *101 Questions Your Brain Has Asked About Itself But Couldn't Answer...Until Now.* 1946. Twenty-First Century Books: Minneapolis, Minnesota.

Calais-Germain, Blandine. *Anatomy of Movement.* 2007. English Language Ed. Eastland Press, Inc.: P.O. Box 99749, Seattle, WA 98139.

Calais-Germain, Blandine. *Anatomy of Movement Exercise,* Revised Edition 2008. Seattle, Washington 98139.

Griswald, Jon. *Beyond Basic Training, Fitness Strategies for Men.* 2003. Saint Martin's Press: New York, New York10010. ISBN 0-312-30755-1.

Hulmes, D. J. S. "Building Collagen Molecules, Fibrils, and Suprafibrillar Structures." *Journal of Structural Biology* 137 (1-2): 2–10. doi:10.1006/jbi.2002.4450. PMID 12064927.

Jarmey, Chris: Thomas W. *The Precise Book of the Moving Body.* ISBN 10.1556436238.

Kornblatt, Sondra. *A Better Brain at Any Age.* "The Holistic Way to Improve Your Memory, Reduce Stress, and Sharpen Your Wits.". 2009. Conari Press: San Francisco, CA.

Krumhardt, Barbara, I. Edward Alcamo. *Baron's E-Z Anatomy and Physiology the Easy Way,* Second Edition. 2004. Barron's Educational Series, Inc.: 251 Wireless Boulevard, Hauppauge, New York, 11788. ISBN-13: 978-0-7641.

Lindsay, David and Anthony A.Vandervoort. "Athletic and Sport Issues in Musculoskeletal Rehabilitation". ISBNO-07-146452-2. *Sports Medicine Board Review,* Second Edition 2006. Richasrd Birrer, Mary Catalelo, Bernarde Griesemer. McGraw-Hill, Medical Publishing Division. Lib. Cong. Catalogue: 2009053345.

Long, Ray, MD FRCSC, *The Key Muscles of Hatha Yoga.* Volume I: 2005, Second Edition: 2006. Banda Yoga Publications.

he Complete Book of Pilates for Men. 2005.
lishers, Inc.: 10 E. 53rd Street, NY 10022. ISBN

luman Body: A Visual Guide. 2006. Firefly Books,
ork.

Murakami, Cathleen. *Morning Pilates Workouts.* 1957. Human Kinetics: Champaign, Illinois, 61825–5076.

Smith, L.K., Weiss, E.L. & Lehmkuhl, L.D. *Brumstrom's Clinical Kinesiology,* Fifth Edition. 1996. F.A. Davis Company: Philadelphia, Pennsylvania.

Organizations and Web Sites

The Human Mind Explained, An Owner's Guide to the Mysteries of the Mind. General Editor Susan A. Greenfield. "Food for Thought" 66–67, "Being Aware" 158–59. 1996. Henry Holt and Company, Inc.: New York, New York.

The Muscular System, Edited by Amy Adams. "Anatomy of the Muscular System" 1–21, "Early Discoveries in Muscle Anatomy and Physiology" 77–99. 2004. Greenwood Press: Westport, CT.

Scripps Physical Therapy Center
Attention of: Alan Ferrarelli, Manager of Rehabilitation Services
9191 Towne Center Drive, Suite 105
San Diego, California 92122

Egosque
Headquarters and Egosque University
12707 High Bluff Drive. Suite 150
San Diego, California 92130

Internet Sources

http://www. Electrophysiology. Cardiac Electrophysiology

http://www. Human Body, Three Planes of Movement

http://www. Phyorg.com "Attention, Couch Potatoes!" Walking boosts brain connectivity, function. University of Illinois at Urbana (Used in Chapter Six)

http://www. Weekly Journal, April 24, 2000, "On Target", Health Newsletter from Target Health, Inc. (Used in Chapter Six)

Science Daily is an online source for topical science articles. It features articles on a wide variety of science subjects including: astronomy, computer science, nanotechnology, medicine, etc.

Elaborations on Research Used in Squared Away

Professors Kramer and McAuley along with their collaborators had 59 sedentary volunteers, age 60 through 79 were divided into three groups: (1) perform aerobic exercise — brisk walking — (2) non-aerobic stretching and toning (3) or nothing for six months. The first two groups started with 15 minutes of exercise and worked up to 45 minutes three times a week. Fitness was monitored and intensity increased as the study progressed.

High-resolution magnetic resonance imaging (MRI) was used, to measure brain volume at the beginning and end of the six-month program. The stretchers-and-toners and the no-exercisers showed no change. The (1) aerobic exercise group, however, showed a significant increase in brain volume. "The prefrontal [memory and attention] and temporal cortices [connects right and left hemispheres] are areas that show considerable age-related deterioration. They incurred the greatest gains from aerobic exercise," reported in the News Bureau.

"After only three months," Professor Kramer told the Wall Street Journal that..."the people who exercised had the brain volume of people three years younger." "This is a great emerging story," said Fred Gage of the Salk Institute, La Jolla, CA, who led the 1998 discovery that humans can grow new brain cells. He added, "You *can* do something to influence your mental fate as you get older."

Another source written by Sharon Begley..."the first time, scientists have found something that not only halts the brain shrinkage that starts in a person's 40s, especially in regions responsible for memory and higher cognition, but actually reverses it." While the 2003 study showed a slowing of the decline in brain density, the new study shows restoration of lost brain volume.

The details are explained by the News Bureau of the University of Illinois at Urbana-Champaign in a release dated November 20, 2006. Additional remarks appeared in *Journal of Gerontology:* MEDICAL SCIENCES, 2006, Vol. 61A, No.11, 1166–1170. Copyright 2006 by The Gerontological Society of America.

17261001R10100

Made in the USA
Lexington, KY
04 September 2012